RESEARCH HIGHLIGHTS
IN SOCIAL WORK

DEVELOPING SERVICES FOR THE ELDERLY

RESEARCH HIGHLIGHTS IN SOCIAL WORK

DEVELOPING SERVICES FOR THE ELDERLY

Second Edition

St. Martin's Press
New York

Editor: Joyce Lishman (with Gordon Horobin)
Secretary: Margaret Donald
Editorial Adviser: Professor G. Rochford

University of Aberdeen
Department of Social Work
King's College
Aberdeen

St. Martin's Press, Inc., 175 Fifth Avenue, New York, N.Y. 10010

Printed in Great Britain

First published in the United States of America in 1985
Library of Congress Catalog Card Number 85-40082

ISBN 0-312-19715-2

LIST OF CONTENTS

Contributors

Joyce Lishman Acting Editor. Ph.D. research at Aberdeen University which explores the relationship between a social worker's prognosis, subsequent behaviour to the client and outcome. Previously a social worker in child and adolescent psychiatry. Publications include 'A Clash in Perspective? A Study of Worker and Client Perceptions of Social Work'. *British Journal of Social Work* 8, 3, 1974 a study of her own practice.

Winifred Rushforth Born in 1885, educated in Edinburgh at the Edinburgh Medical College for Women, graduating in 1908 as M.B., Ch.B. of Edinburgh University. After a year's experience in general practice, she left for India, where she spent the next 20 years, first as a doctor in a mission hospital, largely practising surgery and midwifery, and later, in health education, and in early beginnings of child guidance. Dr. Rushforth married in India in 1915, had four children and is now a matriarch with eleven grandchildren and eleven great-grandchildren. Her interests in psychology began in Calcutta in relationship to people in difficulty and, when she returned to Britain in 1929, she was able to train in psycho-analytic work at the Tavistock Clinic under Dr. Hugh Crichton-Miller. With her husband and children she settled in Edinburgh, and continued in therapeutic practice. In 1939, she set up the Davidson Clinic of which she remained Honorary Medical Director for 25 years. In spite of her age, Dr. Rushforth has continued to carry on work in the analytic field. Group analytic work has developed during the last few years, and this still engages her attention with six such groups meeting weekly under her guidance.

Michael King Lecturer in the Department of Social Work, University of Aberdeen in Residential and Day Care social work. Previous experience includes work as a housefather and housemaster with disturbed children. Work as a generic training officer in Hammersmith. Residential manager, London Borough of Hackney.

David Goda — Research Fellow in the Department of Social Administration, University of Edinburgh. He recently began a study, sponsored by SHHD, of pathways into and between services for the elderly in Scotland. Earlier work, funded by SWSG, included an examination of the available statistics of services for the elderly and a study of training centres for mentally handicapped adults. After lecturing in statistics at Aberdeen University, he was from 1972 until 1977 a statistician in SWSG, where he was closely involved in the design and implementation of the 'Martin' system of social work statistics.

Mark Abrams — Formerly Director of Survey Unit at Social Science Research Council. Now Director of Research Unit at Age Concern. Currently employed on a longitudinal study of ageing in four towns. Recent publications include Alice Foley Annual Memorial Lecture, *Education and the Elderly,* given to WEA, Feb. 1980; *Education in Later Life,* Adult Education Conference - Bolton, Feb. 1981.

Siobhan Lloyd — Lectures in Social Policy and Community Work in the Department of Social Work, University of Aberdeen. Formerly a community worker in Speke, Liverpool and with Merseyside Council for Voluntary Service.

Hans M. Wirz — Senior Lecturer in Department of Social Administration, Edinburgh University. Author of: *Social Aspects of Planning in New Towns* - Saxon House/Teakfield. Editor of *Social Policy Research Monograph Series* for Research Studies Press/Wileys (Titles include: Bruce: 'Teamwork for Preventive Care', Hunter, 'Coping with Uncertainty - Policy and Politics in the National Health Service', and Duncan, 'Low Pay - Its Causes, and the Post-War Trade Union Response'.

Gerard Rochford	Professor of Social Work Studies at Aberdeen University. Previous research and publications in language disorders, professional ethics, the concept of self, and sibling relationships. Most recent publication 'Love, care, control and punishment' in the *Journal of Family Therapy*, 3, 1981. Currently undergoing analytic psychotherapy training through the Scottish Institute of Human Relations.
Barbara Firth	Practice Teacher with Voluntary Service Aberdeen, supervising students in residential, day-care and field-work settings. Formerly Senior Social Worker with the same organisation leading two teams of social workers, one specialising in work with the elderly and the other in Intake work. A large part of this included liaising with the agency's Homes for the Elderly. Previous experience includes social worker on an Intake Team in the London Borough of Waltham Forest.
Cherry Rowlings	Has worked in child care and in post Seebohm intake teams. She was a member of the research team directed by Professors Olive Stevenson and Phyllida Parsloe which studied social work in the local authority and she has a particular interest in work with old people. Currently a lecturer in social work at the University of Bristol, she is also completing a research project on the organisation of social services for physically disabled clients and the role of staff in specialist adviser posts for disability. Cherry Rowlings is a co-author of *Social Service Teams: The Practitioner's View* (DHSS 1978) and author of *Social Work with Elderly People* (Allen and Unwin 1981).
Norma Macleod	Director of Social Work Western Isles Islands Council.
Malcolm Smith	Area Officer (Lewis and Harris) Western Isles Islands Council.

Preface to the Second Edition

The first edition was published in the Spring of 1982. Not surprisingly the issues with which the earlier collection was concerned have not changed but the authors have taken the opportunity to bring their bibliographies up to date. These new references appear under the original chapter headings and Figure 1 and Table 3 of David Goda's paper on 'Relevant Statistics' have also been revised and corrected. The final part of Norma McLeod's and Malcolm Smith's chapter has been more substantially revised.

Some important new research has been initiated since 1982. Particularly worthy of mention are:

1. The 'Informal Care and Support' project in Aberdeen funded mainly by Age Concern, Scotland, which attempts to evaluate the effectiveness of community development workers in mobilising local, informal support for the elderly. (Principal research worker – Dr. David Gordon.) Other research on 'networking' and 'patch' work is being undertaken in Dinnington by Michael Bayley and colleagues.
2. 'Care Delivery Systems for the Elderly'. This is a major cross-national project aimed at identifying the blockages in pathways into and through services especially those associated with separately administered organisations operating on different definitions of need and eligibility. The project is sponsored by the Medical Research Committee of the European Commission and by governmental agencies of the participating countries: Belgium, Denmark, Eire, France, FRG, Greece, Netherlands and U.K. One of the U.K. projects, which has been running for two years, examines pathways through services in North Grampian, Dundee and Forth Valley. (Unit for the Study of the Elderly, Department of Community Medicine, University of Aberdeen; Director: Dr. David Hunter.)

3. The MRC study of 'normal ageing' has already produced some important findings. The research examines *inter alia* the extent of disadvantage and risk to health and psychological functioning of a sample of over 600 elderly people living in their own homes. When compared with the sample as a whole, the isolated, widowed, childless and the poor were not at greater risk of illness or breakdown, whereas the groups at greatest risk were those who had recently moved home, recently been discharged from hospital, were divorced or separated, or were aged over 80. (R. Taylor, G. Ford & H. Barber, 'The Elderly at Risk' *Research Perspectives on Ageing, No. 6* Age Concern Research Unit, 1983.)

These are just a few of the newer research projects aimed at improving understanding of the needs of the elderly, evaluating the different forms of care which are available and highlighting the gaps and overlaps in provision. It would be comforting if one could believe that this burgeoning of research on the elderly will be paralleled by a burgeoning of efficient and effective provision. Forlorn hope or not, a future, completely re-written issue of *Research Highlights* on *Developing Services for the Elderly* may well be needed by 1990.

Editorial

Joyce Lishman

What are the themes of this issue of *Research Highlights?*

Research about the elderly is of personal relevance to us all: we are all likely to grow old. It is equally of professional relevance: Goda's paper shows dramatically the projected increase in the elderly as a proportion of the population, and Rowlings quotes from a Grampian Social Work Department report, 'Already half of the Social Work Department revenue budget is spent on care of the elderly'.

What does it mean to be old? It is difficult to generalise about the elderly when 35 years separates the oldest from the youngest (Abrams). Cultural and ideological differences affect the status of the elderly. Stereotyping leads to public expectations of illness, isolation, and deprivation which exceed the experience of the elderly themselves (King).

Poverty is a likely concomitant of old age, although there is considerable inequality of income and expenditure among the elderly. Poverty is socially generated: the elderly are expected and indeed generally forced not to work, and to be dependent on the state. Yet the assumption of our society is that those who do not work should be worse off than those who do. Thus loss of income leads to loss of status (King).

Dealing with loss is one of the tasks of old age; loss of income, work and status have already been referred to. The elderly also face the increased possibility of loss of health, of house and independent living, of important people, and, in time, the final loss - of their own lives, death.

'Good Health', is important to the elderly themselves (Abrams). *New Scientist*[1] recently summarising a Dutch survey of disablement in the EEC points out that the problem of disabled people is a problem of age;

for people between 5 and 24 only 2% are handicapped whereas for the over 75s the proportion rises to 35%.

Loss of one's own house and consequently independent living contributes to anxiety about becoming old. The number of elderly people living alone has increased and as a group the elderly often live in the worst housing (Wirz). There is an association between inadequate housing, and anxiety and clinical depression. Add to this poverty and ill health, and maintaining independent living becomes impossible (Rowlings).

Finally, old age is often associated with isolation, loss of contact with others, and with bereavement; spouse, siblings, friends, even children are more likely to die as one ages (Rochford).

Here then are some of the problems of old age, and particularly of extreme old age. However old age should not be seen as inevitably constituting a problem, as Winifred Rushforth so clearly exemplifies. Some of the problems of old age are culturally and socially created.

How do the services respond? Rowlings raises the question of definition of need, complicated by the difference between felt need (not necessarily expressed) and expressed need, a particular problem for the bereaved (Rochford).

Money is the greatest need; Lloyd's paper raises the possibility of index-linking of pensions, but more fundamentally questions the present effect of the relationship between age, the labour market and reward for work.

Wirz looks at the use of sheltered housing and concludes that on the basis of satisfaction of the elderly it is highly successful, although only serving a very small minority. Regrettably this edition lacks a paper reviewing research on health service provision to the elderly, hospital and community. Readers will certainly be aware of gaps in this provision and problems of definition of responsibility between medical and social work services. Rochford's paper draws upon the literature on bereavement counselling and its implications for developing services for the elderly.

Residential care affects only a small proportion of the elderly (Goda). Firth's paper on residential care highlights the gaps in research there: the lack of criteria for good and bad practice, the problem of models of care being posed with no comparative research on how they actually work, and the problem of how to differentiate elderly client groups and match with appropriate care. The majority of the elderly, however, remain in the community. Rowlings focusses on the care of dementing parents by their family, and supports for the careers e.g. granny sitting, relief holidays, day care, which are relevant not just to dementia but more generally to families caring for the old at home. Macleod and Smith in their practice model, describe one authority's organisation of 'formal' care (home helps, day care, relief wardens) to support the elderly and their carers, to enable old people to continue to live in the community.

The last two papers raise the issue of the relationship between formal and informal care. Bayley[2] explored the extent to which an organised service structured and organised itself to mesh in with and support informal care (interweaving). Neighbourhood schemes and volunteers or paid workers (e.g. street wardens, or the home helps and wardens in a patch system)[3] can attempt to provide the caring which might be carried out by natural helping networks. However Barker[4] questions the focus on a good neighbour and refers instead to the need for friendship, and intimacy for old people's survival. He suggests old people prefer informal help fom an intimate because professional help provided by formal agencies is seen as labelling oneself as a problem or deviant or disabled, whereas informal help is reciprocal and a normal part of life. In his view, this intimate would then be the key person to whom the formal services referred.

Further, since reviews of past research[5] indicate that 'spontaneous' caring networks of neighbours and friends are the exception, even if the family is the major source of personal services and care, is the emphasis on informal care realistic? Nevertheless to rely on formal care entirely seems more unrealistic in terms of provision and acceptability to the elderly. From the carer's point of view the costs of informal care are high[6].

If informal care is seen as an essential ingredient in providing for the elderly, research is needed to discover more about its nature and networks, and how to support them. In practice, social workers need also to be aware of its nature, and ensure that formal services are organised round informal care rather than organising it.

This issue draws together research on need among the elderly and the provision of services for them. It is difficult to summarise but three conclusions stand out:

1. the importance of consistency in assessment of need,
2. the importance of differentiating need and matching provision accordingly, e.g. for one old person beset with anxiety about frailty, poverty and housing, residential care may provide welcome relief: another's

anxiety may be lessened by the support of a home help and the reassurance of continuing in home and community,

3. the importance of evaluating service provision and establishing criteria for doing this, including cost, ease of administration but most important, satisfaction of the old person.

REFERENCES:

1. 'Just who are the disabled'? *New Scientist*, 26 Nov. 1981, p. 593.
2. Bayley, M. *Community Orientated Systems of Care*. Unpublished Paper.
3. Shanon, H. 'A Stitch in Time' in *Social Work Today*, V, 13, No. 18, 12:1:82.
4. Barker, J. "The Relationship of 'Informal' Care to 'Formal' Social Services: Who helps people deal with social and health problems if they arise in old age"? in *Teamwork in Personal Social Services and Health Care* (Eds.) Lonsdale, S., Webb, A. & Briggs, J. Croom Helm & Syracuse University, School of Social Work, N.Y. 1980.
5. Abrams, P. 'Community Care: Some Research Problems and Priorities' in *Policy and Politics*, 6, 2, December 1977.
6. Nissel, M. & Bonnerjea, L. *Family Care of the Handicapped Elderly: Who Pays?* Policy Studies Institute, 112 Castle Lane, London, SW1.

The editor wishes to acknowledge the assistance of Mr. A. Murray (Co-ordinator : Grampian Regional Social Work Department) in thinking about the relationship of formal and informal care.

Introduction

Winifred Rushforth

When men and women come into their forties, the fifth decade of their lives, they are likely to find that younger friends look on them as elderly. When I was about forty, a lass in her twenties referred to 'old people like you and your husband'. Soon afterwards I found the following 'Thought for the Day':

> "Men should know we are growing old not by the frailty of the body but by the strength and creativity of the spirit".

Now many years have passed and a wise friend writes urging me to value the tenth decade of my life. He affirms that most old people who have lived their life well, (by which he means have lived in loving relationship with their fellows) will have opportunities in quite unconscious ways to bring blessings into the community.

How can we 'live well' and maintain the energy which keeps us from ageing?

Let us think of ourselves as foursquare: Jung refers to the four functions which if integrated into our personality make us whole people. Two of these functions, intuition and sensation, belong to all living things. Intuition is awareness, knowing without the intervention of thought. Sensation is contact with the environment through the body, in human touching, hearing, seeing, smelling, tasting. As life develops through evolution the contact between parent and offspring leads to the development of the feeling function. At first it is the awakening of tenderness - a bird gathers her chicks under her wing while attacking the intruder who would interfere with her brood. Reptiles and fish also lay eggs but with them there is no development of tenderness, since they keep no contact with their young. Love is dependent on this contact at the beginning of life. So vulnerable and probably so fear-ridden is the emergent creature that of necessity the parents must shelter and protect it and also defend it against the onslaught of enemies. Mammals and marsupials show the same feelings which in human beings we recognise as love and hate.

The fourth function, that of thought, is peculiar to mankind. The human forebrain with its capacity to reason, to choose, to make decisions, has developed through thousands of years replacing thc olfactory lobes of the four-footed mammals. They keep their noses close to the ground and are guided by smell, of which only weak traces survive in present day man.

Man's ability to think and reason has led to a vast accumulation of knowledge: a great world of Science has been built up and has led to every kind of human activity involving tools and instruments, from Adam's spade to the Palimar Observatory and the nuclear bomb. These are the result of humanity's gift for thinking function. But thought and rationality can so easily be at the expense of the earlier, more primitive functions of life, bringing a crippling loss in the personality of the individual. It is the cultivation of our four-sidedness that enables us to grow into maturity of spirit that makes light of the inevitable decrease in bodily strength.

In order to grow old wisely, cheerfully, without regrets, I suggest that we do not allow ourselves to give up the use and the enjoyment of our four-sidedness. Intuition is likely to persist longer than reason as it has roots so deep in life. Under the name of the 'hunch' it is common to all and we should not lightly discard it but rather trust our hunches even at times giving them precedence over rational knowledge. In old age, with failing memory and diminished ability to see and hear, we can keep this inner wisdom of the psyche, sharing it as we do with young children and primitive people.

Sensation too may be cultivated even with failing eyesight or hearing. The hand with its delicate fingers need never lose pleasure in contact with rough things or smooth. A firm grasp makes for safety and we can express much love and tenderness by touch and gesture. Is it only our imagination that makes us find the scent of roses and honeysuckle ever increasingly a joy?

What of the heart, our ability to feel? It is sad that modern, 'civilised' life patterns have tended to deny the value of feeling, putting great emphasis on the need to think. Feeling values are repressed as unacceptable when children are told to keep a stiff upper lip. Boys in particular are discouraged from weeping and are labelled as soft and girlish. Professional women, too, are warned against letting their feelings get the upper hand.

Young nurses in our hospitals are, all too often, told that there is no time to waste in giving sympathy to their patients. I well remember a dream that came to me when I was beginning to understand the conflict between the heart and the intellect. In my dream I was aboard a great liner on its way from Bombay to London passing through the Straits of Messina. We had ploughed through the depths of the Indian Ocean and the Red Sea. We had found the Suez Canal adequate to take the great ship, and the Mediterranean held us safely in its depths. Now we were approaching Marseilles where I would disembark, soon finding myself in London again committed to professional duties. As I watched, in the dream, from the prow of the ship I was horrified to see the shallowness of the water. Since in the dream water symbolises feeling, I took the dream as a powerful warning not to sacrifice feeling and become immersed in thinking, learning and professional work. It was a great influence in my life since I was just beginning the experience and practise of psychoanalysis and needed to remember that in *straitened* circumstances we must depend on feeling rather than on thought.

Finally, what of the fourth function, thought? It is the last to be developed in the course of evolution and for that reason vulnerable. A blow on the head, a glass too much alcohol and we are incapable of thought. Intense emotion is likely to deprive us of our ability to think: we become instead in a state of panic, infatuation or suffering.

Since my focus is on the ageing process and the question, 'need the psyche deteriorate because the bodily physique is weakening'? we must keep in mind the four-squaredness and endeavour to maintain the use of all four functions throughout our lives. Let us consider then how best we can maintain and possibly increase our use of the closing years. Let me share with you what I have learned as I now approach a century. Undoubtedly we must take acocunt of our genetic inheritance as well as our earthly nature and realise that some of us human beings are more gifted with one or other of these four capacities; intuition, sensation, feeling and thought. But this need not be a reason for envy or despair, but rather a determination to use and cultivate as much as possible in our personalities for as long as possible.

In order the develop *intuition* at any stage of life, we should learn to become more aware and more trustful of our hunches. We might tell someone about it when they come true, or even keep a notebook to record them. In any case if we trust our hunches, we shall undoubtedly discover that they are trust-worthy.

To maintain the *sensation* function my advice would be 'Keep your hand in', by which we mean that no skill should be lost prematurely for lack of use. Cooking, gardening, knitting, music making, painting, sketching can all be practised in old age.

To maintain the *heart* function deliberately and consciously we can decide to practise 'the law of love' which involves us in the giving and taking of relationships. Our old friends die and there is of necessity a sense of loss but through my own experience I can testify that to give love brings love. Gestures, words, deeds that you can still use, however old you may be, will bring great reward in friendship. We need not hold to the childish ideas about 'best friend' and so on. An individual life broadens and flows when it is devoted to the care of others. We should know ourselves as conduits, through which psychic energy can flow from the Source into the life of humanity. I quote some beautiful words from the Apocryphal book of Ecclesiasticus:

> 'I go to water my orchard, to irrigate my flower beds, see the conduit has become a river and the river a sea'.

How best can we maintain the most recent function, our *thinking*? We must endeavour to keep in contact with ideas through books and through talking to people, always being ready to consider ideas that are not immediately acceptable.

Good teachers and wise parents encourage their pupils and avoid discouragement. Age involves actual loss of brain cells; in consequence the process of *learning*, that is the capacity to acquire new knowledge, slows down with the passing of years. To learn a poem committing it to memory, can be a simple and easy task in schooldays, but increasingly difficult in old age although not impossible. To overcome the difficulty and find oneself still able to acquire fresh passages of poetry or prose in memory brings great pleasure and to make a habit of this may well retard the process of memory deterioration that is so wounding to one's self respect. The admission of the 'mature student' to our Universities and the recent establishment of the Open University are opening up great possibilities for people no longer young.

If we expect great things of ourselves and others, even in old age we shall be rewarded. In his teaching on auto-suggestion Coué insisted that we should avoid the use of the negative but always make positive statements. For instance, at bedtime, if we avoid the *not* in 'I shall not wake up tired in the morning' and say instead 'I shall wake up as fresh as paint in the morning' our minds are likely to heed and the body to respond. By making a habit of this way of thinking and talking we can establish an optimism affecting not only ourselves but also others whom our lives touch. Whether or not we attain a 'Happy Old Age' must to a very great extent depend on our ability to relate to our neighbours caringly, to regard ourselves well, and to live in the here and now without anticipation of trouble ahead, but with faith always that *ALL WILL BE WELL*.

Review of the Literature and Gaps

Michael King

INTRODUCTION

All of us are growing older. We know, if our health holds out, we suffer no serious accidents, and there are no nuclear catastrophes, we shall reach the age of 65. An increasing number will survive to the age of 85. Currently 15% of the United Kingdom population, approximately 8 million people, are 65 years or over. Most demographic projections indicate that this figure will increase and so also will the number surviving 85.[1] There will be a ratio of three women to every man. This paper aims to look at what research can tell us about the future of the elderly, with particular reference to Scotland.

INTERNATIONAL RESEARCH

Cargill and Holmes[2] studied ageing in fourteen different societies, ranging from the primitive to modern society. In all the countries studied they found the aged were a minority, females outnumbered males, and widowhood was highly represented. Old people tend to shift from active economic productive roles to sedentary advisory and supervisory roles. All the societies tended to have some elderly politicians, judges and leaders, and their customs tended to prescribe mutual responsibility between old people and their adult children. All the societies valued life and tried to prolong it.

However the societies studied classify and accordingly treat old people differently. In unmodernised societies people were classified as old at a younger age, and this was more likely to be related to status than chronological age. The status of the aged was high in unmodernised agricultural societies, characterised by extended families, where the aged occupy more powerful positions, particularly if they are valued and useful. There is no retirement in unmodernised societies.

ELDERLY PEOPLE IN INDUSTRIAL SOCIETIES[2]

In modern industrialised societies the status of the aged is different: it is more clearly related to chronological age. People tend to live longer and societies include a higher proportion of women and widows, of grandparents and great grandparents. The status of the elderly in modern societies seems to be lower if there is rapid social change, and if they live in urban rather than agricultural communities. It decreases with the increased literacy of a society. Retirement is a recent phenomena of modern societies. Status decreases within nuclear families, and in societies where the newly married are relocated away from the parental home. The numbers of elderly who are in leadership roles decreases in modern societies. The individualistic value system of western society tends adversly to affect the security and status of older people. The more modern the society the more the tendency for the elderly to disengage or be disengaged is noted. In general older people retain their status and self respect if they continue to fulfil a useful function in society. Power may confer status and respect on the elderly person, but it does not always command affection.

Interesting exceptions in industrialised societies occur in the case of Russia and Poland where elderly people have retained relatively higher status than in the West. It had been suggested by Cargill and Holmes[2] that this is partly because of a collectivist rather than an individualist philosophy and because of elderly people's greater relative wealth and mobility, eligibility for a pension and access to free public services.

THE ELDERLY IN EUROPE - A CROSS CULTURAL VIEW

One study[3] *Open Care for the Elderly in Seven European Countries: a pilot study in the Possibilities and Limits of Care,* has examined Austria, Denmark, Greece, Hungary, the Netherlands, Poland and Yugoslavia. The countries vary not only in their degree of industrialisation but also in proportion of their elderly population (i.e.) 20.2% are over 65+ in Denmark compared with 12.2% in Yugoslavia. Europe, generally has seen the proportion of elderly people increase from 10 to 15% to 15 to

20% in the last twenty years and this figure would have been much higher if the population had not suffered war losses. The maximum point of 'the explosion' of the elderly has already been reached in some countries and it is not seen as a group that will mushroom for ever as some studies suggest.

In Europe, elderly women seem the most disadvantaged. They live longer, are disadvantaged in terms of status in society, more likely than men to lose a spouse, and suffer all the economic disadvantages of widowhood. In Europe, general assistance is concentrated in connurbations while remaining underdeveloped in rural areas and small municipalities.

The links between the system of social services have been highlighted in two United Nations reports. [4]

1. Social services may supplement social security services and cash benefits complementing each other to maintain the recipient's independence (e.g.) home helps, meals on wheels.
2. Social services may strengthen social security benefits (e.g.) giving welfare rights information.
3. Social services may substitute for social security in cases where security payments are totally insufficient and when the individual cannot live independently at home even with community and domiciliary help.

Whose responsibility: the family's or society's?[3]

Both in Yugoslavia where the needs of the aged are becoming the problem of the whole society not just the family, and in the Netherlands, statutory and voluntary assistance is increasing, although the family is still important at least in identifying the needs of their elderly and organising and alerting services to meet their needs. In all countries the family remains a source of help, particularly in terms of the work done by female relatives. Only in Greece is the family entirely central, whereas other countries ambivalently seek separation and involvement of the family with their relatives at different times, although it remains a refuge in emergencies.

European countries have developed their notions of care of the elderly according to individual ideologies e.g. religious, socio-economic, and political perspectives. In the Eastern block ideology governs income maintenance and pension schemes, so that farmers are often relatively deprived and civil servants relatively prosperous.

PROBLEMS FOR THE ELDERLY

[1] *Poverty*

Whereas pensions used to be viewed as social protection for old age, they are now viewed increasingly as wage replacement. In Europe many elderly people find the pensions they receive on retirement are less than their earnings causing a substantial drop in their living standards and the experience of relative poverty. In Austria the old age pension of a blue collar worker in 1975 was 38.6% of the average *per capita* income of all employed. Thus other schemes are introduced to supplement the elderly person's inability to survive on a pension well below the poverty line (e.g.) rent rebates, subsidised transport, rate rebates. One indication of the increasing poverty of the elderly is whereas formerly the pattern was that parents helped children financially, Strieb's study[5] showed that now the more elderly the parents and the less income they had, the more likely were the children to care for the parents in cash and kindness. In recent years percentage contact frequency between children and other parents remained high: 88% of old people in Poland, 82% in Great Britain, 77% in the United States and 75% in Denmark have children living no more than half an hour's walking distance away. However, we do not know the quality of family relationships, the effect of supporting a poor parent, or the degree of reluctance that elderly parents have in requesting help from their children who often have family commitments.

In most countries pensions are index-linked, yet are falling behind the average wage although less in socialist countries. In Poland the plan was to fix pensions at 80% of previous earning level, although this was not index-linked and recent doubling of food prices must have reduced the real value of pensions.

A Dutch General Pension Act has been considered to ensure a pension of 70% of previous earnings.

Amann[3] has shown that old people in disadvantaged situations tend to shift their expectations downwards over time, ceasing to look for better accommodation and make plans for the future or holidays.

[2] *Health*

In the Netherlands and Nordic countries home help and nursing are an integral part of community care. In Denmark a home nursing system is mandatory for local authorities. In the Netherlands, where 13.7% of elderly people live in institutions, including 10% in residential homes, the policy is to reduce this to 7%. The health services in the Netherlands do not favour specialised medical services for the elderly, but advocate their incorporation into the general health system. Health support for the elderly is performed in most countries by the general practitioner, social welfare homes, and by voluntary societies.

While most elderly people in Europe and Britain do not suffer from malnutrition, there is a connection in the minority of old people who do between isolation, depression, poverty and state of health.[3] The same study points to substantial evidence, that the bare subsistence level of many of the elderly results in poor health. Low income results in low protein diets, and bad diets in low resistance to hypothermia.

[3] *Housing*

Amann's[3] survey of the elderly in Europe indicates the importance of accommodation for the elderly in that old people spend an increasing amount of time in their homes. However the living environment does not end at the four walls of the home, but includes access to transport, shops, medical services and recreation.

[4] *Isolation and Desolation*

Townsend and Tunstall[6] referred to infrequent social relationships as *isolation* and the grief and apathy following the sudden loss of a long standing close relationship as *desolation*, resulting in a kind of emotional depression.

Club membership is one way of breaking down isolation, but tends not to be used often by those not used to clubs in their earlier life. One resource which might be tapped is the elderly person himself. Amann has indicated that much of what is being done *for* the elderly could also be done *by* and *with* the elderly and gives examples of people in their 70s and 80s who have been active, e.g. in painting , Picasso and in philosophy, Russell.

CARE POLICY IN EUROPE[3]

European countries describe their residential homes, nursing homes and hospitals, as closed care, while open care consists of day centres, health centres, domiciliary services, clubs and associations for the elderly. The family is also seen as a type of open care. Open/closed care provides day care in residential centres, offering respite to relatives and friends. In the Netherlands, 10% of the elderly people live in institutions while Yugoslavia has less than 1%.

Day Care for the elderly varies widely in Europe. In Denmark, meals on wheels and luncheon clubs exist. *Respite care* allowing relatives to go on holiday exists in the form of temporary relief accommodation, while some nursing homes have full-time and day-time residents. 'Day time homes for a week' allow people in rural areas to spend the nights at the home as well as the days, (since rural areas are not generally as well resourced with residential homes as urban areas). This also tends to make closed homes more open.

In Hungary old people can spend the long winter evenings and nights at a centre to counter depression and loneliness. In Poland a number of elderly people take their midday meal in the cafeteria of their former work place.

In Denmark, home helps are trained: they spend 90% of their time providing help to the elderly in 20% of households of the elderly. In Austria, only Vienna boasts a well-developed home help service. In other parts social work aides provide home help on an emergency basis. Problems home helps must guard against are the creation of dependency arising from services provided, and the tendency for the family to withdraw.

In the Netherlands day care includes the provision of service centres which offer social, cultural and leisure activities, physiotherapy, occupational therapy, pedicure, baths, meals, diet advice and social counselling. Day centres also take on post-hospital care, fulfil an alarm-monitoring function, relieve families, and provide a break for the elderly person from their family.

THE ELDERLY IN EUROPE: POLICY IMPLICATIONS AND CONCLUSIONS

Amann[3] argues that to avoid piecemeal development of a favourite service, whether it be home helps or old people's homes - the needs of the elderly have to be satisfied in many different ways simultaneously, including improved sanitation, central heating in homes, mobile health teams, laundry service. Services would be better designed to dovetail rather than reflect policy makers' personal preferences. Community (open) and residential care (closed) are functionally related, less domiciliary and community care means more residential care. Some old people were socialised into conditions of hardship in the past and have low aspirations. The economic and social realities of modern society mean that the old and impaired have little chance of gaining social esteem and power.

WHAT IS IT LIKE TO GROW OLD?

In a poll conducted by the Harris Polling Organisation for the National Council on the Ageing,[7] it was found that younger general public see growing older as more problematic for the elderly, than the elderly themselves. In over 4,250 interviews held with a representative cross section of American adults, the replies indicated that public expectations exceeded that of the elderly themselves. They expected more old people to fear crime, suffer from loneliness, have insufficient education and medical care, not feel needed, not have enough to do, have few friends, not enough job opportunities, live in poor housing and have insufficient clothing. The survey indicated that young adults expected the above problems to be more severe than they are for the elderly who actually experience them. However these problems do exist for a real minority of elderly people.

Harris and his associates[7] found in their survey that income and racial background have been identified as having a greater impact on life satisfaction than does age. Hendricks & Hendricks[8] assert that the realities of ageing do not fit the stereotypes: most of the elderly are not isolated, ill, emotionally distraught or bereaved by loss of job through retirement. Elderly women are not traumatised by the loneliness of the empty nest, nor are elderly people sexually inactive or even lacking interest. Undoubtedly it is difficult to generalise since there are obvious exceptions. But from research the irony emerges that while the young may see the elderly as having more problems than they admit they experience, the elderly may be justified in seeing themselves to be the victims of stereotyping by the young, of being defined as a problem, rather than having a contribution to make in society.

THE SITUATION IN THE UNITED KINGDOM

Old age does not necessarily involve disability and problems and the majority of elderly people do not come into contact with the welfare services. Eighty per cent of elderly people are not physically impaired and 90% are not suffering from mental deterioration nor are the majority confined to the house, wheel chair or bed.[9]

Brearley[10] argues that since only about 5% of old people are in institutional care, and 13% are housebound then 80% live relatively active lives in the community. But this situation is changing, as the older a person gets the more risk of disability, residential care and dependency. Brearley points out that although only a few people receive services at any one time, a growing number can expect to receive services at some time. The anxiety expressed by long term planners to expand services for the elderly in the next twenty years are based on surveys like that of Abrams [11] who suggests that while the numbers of people between 65 and 74 years of age will fall between 1976-1996, the number of those aged 75 and over will increase by three-quarters of a million (23%).

Retirement

Growing older inevitably means in modern industrial societies retiring from employment at a certain age. Palmore[12] suggests that compulsory retirement is by definition age discrimination. He considers it unfair to the capable older worker, psychologically and socially damaging and economically wasteful, resulting in the loss of the elderly person's talents and skills. The alternative to compulsory retirement, much advocated at times of recession, would be shorter working weeks, longer holidays, delayed entry into the labour market and extension of educational opportunities. As I write, the British University, Polytechnic and Higher Education system and the Adult Community Education Classes are being cut. I remember, vividly, studying at an Open University summer school with a 91 year old retired pharmacist who was realising his ambition to read for a degree, for which he had never had time previously. The Open University is also being cut, and as a result has had to increase its fees, effectively prohibiting all but the rich elderly from participating.

Being old and poor

Townsend[13] has suggested that poverty in old age is the outcome of a life long process, so that some old people are poor as a result of the low class position they have always occupied, while others are made poor by relegation to 'an under-class' due to imposed retirement with its lower income. There clearly do exist rich and poor elderly people. The rich elderly may find old age more easily lived in secure privately owned property and with no anxieties about heating, proper diet, transport, due to a good pension buttressed by accumulated capital. The poor elderly may, throughout their life possess a low level of resources, restricted access to education, and job opportunities, while working for basic wages without a chance to progress through a financially attractive career structure. They may have always rented accommodation in either the public or private sector. People occupying low status jobs, are also more at risk from redundancy, and unemployment, and from occupational injury and resulting disability. Poor elderly people, on retirement, are likely to rely for their livelihood on the state social security system. Growing older, frequently means seeing spending power diminishing, seeing the value of carefully saved money eroded through inflation. Widowhood means the loss of the expected support of a work pension. The elderly also live in ageing property and the chances are that while the younger working family might have resources to install central heating, the elderly person on a pension will not. In 1971, 76% of heads of household aged 65 and over (and 82% of the over 80s) were in homes without central heating while 57% of heads of household aged 25 - 44 had central heating.[14]

Being old and alone

Growing older, inevitably means having fewer friends or relatives as they die with increasing rapidity, or their children move away to seek new employment opportunities. Current government policy conveys a dual message, encouraging younger people to be mobile and seek work on the one hand, while also insisting that it is the duty of the family to care for its elderly on the other, (i.e. stay with them). The elderly rapidly become victims of the work ethic, that espouses job mobility, job efficiency, and greater productivity for the young. This is made more critical by the relocation of populations due to property speculation, gentrification of old working class areas, and the inevitable separation of the young, displaced to new towns to meet the needs of new industries, while their parents are left in decaying inner city areas.

PROFESSIONAL HELP FOR THE ELDERLY

This involves several questions: how need/demand for help is to be assessed, what help then best meets the needs and what is the shortfall in existing help. The study, *Needs of the Elderly in the Scottish Borders*[15] makes the point that the elderly have needs, but because most do not tend to translate their needs to the point of demanding services, they are missed by the professionals. Need must be defined before it can be measured. This survey was commissioned by the Borders Region with a view to implementing estimates of need, in services. At the time of the survey four councils, two executive councils and two hosipital boards of management had responsibilities for the elderly and the rate of provision of hospital beds, domiciliary services and residential placements varied widely over the constituent authorities. It was discovered that both provision and utilisation of services was interpreted differently by different bodies at an administrative and personal level, with the consequent likelihood of unmet need.

Method

A register was compiled from GP files of people over 65. They were then sampled by age/sex/rural or urban living and GP. Those receiving residential and domiciliary services were included if they fell into the sample. Permission was sought from GPs to make medical records of the sample available. Interviews were conducted to build up a social picture of the lives of the elderly people in the area in terms of social and family contact, standard of housing, ability to perform tasks and their present use of services.

The medical questionnaire attempted to indicate the presence of conditions which might affect the mobility and independence of the elderly and their need for medical attention. Comparisons were then made between the GP's records and the questionnaire.

Findings

The survey found that 61.9% lived in urban areas and 38.1% in rural areas, 36.8% were 65 - 69 years of age, 27.2% between 70 - 74 years of age, and 36.8% over 75. Five per cent of those circulated were too confused to answer the questionnaire.

Ninety-four per cent lived in private households and more than a third had lived in the house for over 20 years. Six per cent had moved in last year and 19.6% between 1 - 5 years ago. Some people tended to move after retirement but usually not very far. Some of those in tied housing had to leave the area on retirement.

Half of those questioned were single or widowed and one third had no living offspring. Of those with children, 26.4% lived in the same household and 62.4% locally. Replies indicated that old people value contact most with their own children and then in descending order of importance; other younger generation relatives, friends, relatives of the same generation, neighbours, minister or priest. One per cent had no visitors at all while 6% had no single visitor for as long as a month.

Most people went out daily but 7% never went out and 5% less than once a month. The most common outings were to relations and shops. Twenty per cent had either full of part-time employment. Nine per cent did voluntary work and 70% had three or more different interests or hobbies.

One third of those questioned lived in houses rented from the local authority. Only 3% were in purpose built accommodation for the elderly and less than 1% in sheltered housing. Twenty per cent lacked one of the basic amenities. Sixty-four per cent used only coal fires, some gathering wood from the surrounding countryside. Twenty-four per cent did all their own housework, 72% were helped by relatives and 7% did none. Only 3.9% had home help.

Few were receiving domiciliary services. Two per cent had meals on wheels. Most of those questioned had a positive attitude to the social services and knew about them. Almost a quarter of the elderly had restrictions on going out.

The study showed that rheumatism, psychological symptoms and cardio vascular diseases were the major medical diagnoses in a large proportion of the elderly. Although 47% had not seen their doctor in the last three months, it was still the GP and medical services who carried the biggest load of community care for the elderly and the GP was seen to be the person in the best position to recognise need. When asked what changes would improve their lives, 45% could think of none, 24.6% wanted more money and 17.6% alterations to their houses.

The study shows that 65% of elderly men live with a spouse compared to 29% of women (twice as many women as men have never married) and twice as many are widowed. Twice as many women live alone, but women are visited more frequently than men by a greater variety of people.

Although a similar proportion of men and women had recently been bereaved or had lost contact with someone, 8% of men had recently given up employment and some other regular activity compared to 3% of women. Men tended not to do housework and this was frequently not due to incapacity. Women have a less favourable attitude to social services than men. Fewer women than men had a car although as many women as men have a telephone. Men and women in this survey suffered from the same mean number of medical conditions, but in men respiratory conditions, peptic ulcers, strokes and other neurological conditions were common and in women joint disease, rheumatism, eye conditions and psychological symptoms were more common. Degree of dependence varied little but women had more trouble going out and climbing stairs. Although seen equally frequently by the GP, 42% of women were seen at home compared to 28% of men. Women were also more frequently visited by the nursing services than men.

While as many of the young as old elderly had problems with lack of amenities, increasing age was in general associated with increasing deprivation of all kinds. There is a steep fall in those who have a marriage partner from 60% in the 65 - 70 age category to 14% in those over 80. The proportion of those who never married rises from 15% in those under 75 years to 25% in the 80 + age group.

Forty-three per cent of those over 80 have no living offspring. However older people were more likely to live with their children than the young elderly, involving loss of independence.

The proportion of those in residential homes increases with age although the older a person is the less favourable their attitude to residential care. It was also noted that while feelings of loneliness and lack of things to do increased with age somewhat, feelings of contentment do not.

In terms of social class, all classes have an equal distribution of multiple pathology and are attended to equally by the health services and just as many in each social class were in institutions. No class differences existed in terms of living alone or being visited, and people from various social classes tended to belong to associations their class in general would attend. The differences are that manual workers were more frequently widowed. Classes IV & V had more living offspring, at hand, than other social classes.

None of the professionals lived in sheltered accommodation, and three times as many people from classes IV and V did so than III. Ninety-four per cent of classes I & II had all amenities whereas 26% of III and 27% of IV & V lacked at least one. Only 19% of classes I & II did their own housework compared to 25% in class III and 28% in classes IV & V. Class I tended to hire private help whereas the lower classes received help from their children. Forty-eight per cent of classes I & II were car owners compared to 11% of classes IV & V, while 64% of classes I & II had telephones in their homes compared to 9% of classes IV & V.

Rural areas tend to have a higher proportion of elderly people in classes I and V. Twice as many country people had cars. While fewer country people lived alone, they did have fewer visitors, and there were fewer meals on wheels and home helps.

Those suffering from psychological symptoms had a strong association between social isolation and depression. Those dependent on personal care suffered less from depression and anxiety. Being in an institution with others may also lessen the symptoms. Older age groups and women suffer more psychological symptoms but this could be related to impairment (e.g. depression arising from loss of mobility). Inadequate housing is also linked to the presence of psychological symptoms but not lack of money, social class or rural living.

This study shows that the questionnaire and limited observation found 3.1 conditions (physical and psychological) per person of which 1.2 were not apparently recorded by the GP. Seventy per cent of the sample appeared to have one or more unrecorded condition likely to affect their lives significantly. GPs may not inquire about their conditions which they are not currently treating:

- 15% experienced difficulty in seeing with their spectacles (had not had their eyes tested for over 6 years).
- 19% had difficulty hearing normal speech.
- 4% found their hearing aid unsatisfactory.
- 22% had difficulty in walking but were not receiving physiotherapy.

The study concludes that there does not seem to be any clear definition of the need for social services and researchers have to apply the definition of the local authorities concerned which vary from authority to authority. The proportion spent on social services depend on the controlling local authority. Nor is the role of the family clear in the case of the elderly. There is a considerable subjective element in the allocation of services.

Using this study's criteria (scoring on the anxiety, depression scale, or chronic brain syndrome, in need of money or domestic help, with limited social contact) 58% of the sample were in need of advice and guidance from a social worker, 11% were in need of domestic help and 29% might qualify for more money.

The study suggests three schemes for screening the elderly to identify unmet need. The scheme to screen all elderly would involve a high level of extra manpower; a second scheme might restrict its screening to those over 75 years of age, while a third scheme might look at 'at risk' groups excluding those in a local authority home or hospital. This 'at risk' category would include those living alone, those recently bereaved, those having difficulty with walking, those with evidence of mental impairment and those recently discharged from hospital. By this definition half the elderly population are 'at risk'. Even to screen the over 75s or the 'at risk' group would leave half the needs undetected.

Unmet needs

A non-Scottish report[16] describes an action research project into the unmet needs of a sample of elderly people living in the City of Westminster. The research team attempted not only to uncover unmet needs but also to ensure that those needs for services and benefits were met by the local authority. It was successful in only half the cases. Chapman suggests that for an elderly person to apply for help, a need first had to be felt. He pinpoints two groups whose needs are not met, those who don't recognise they have difficulties, (a small proportion of elderly mentally handicapped or confused people) and those who do not feel a need for help, (who are very aware of their difficulties but prefer to manage on their own or are dissatisfied with services provided).

The report suggested eight major factors which determine the difficulties old people face in expressing their positive need for welfare services.

1. *Publicity of service* - one reason for not publishing may be because of availability in terms of limited resources despite a statutory duty to provide services.
2. *Proliferation of services and benefits*
   In the survey conducted, there were ten welfare services dispensed, administered by six organisations excluding the full range of health services and financial benefits. Some elderly people are confused as to which body or department to contact.
3. *Application procedures*
   To apply for all services made few active demands on elderly people

and in general there is little form filling. In spite of this many elderly people are unsure about how to apply or whether they are eligible, and may therefore be deterred from applying.

4. *Control by gatekeepers*
Friends, welfare officials and GPs play an important role as providers of information and contact between old people and welfare services, and it has been asserted that they protect welfare services from demands which would otherwise be made on them. Welfare officials and GPs often underrate the needs of elderly clients compared to the old people themselves.
5. *Psychological factors*
Reports indicate overall intellectual ability declines with age and may affect an elderly person's ability to report his need. It is mainly short term memory that suffers with ageing. Many people claim to be able to manage even when a need is felt, and require encouragement to apply for services they clearly need.
6. *Physical health*
Although the majority of old people are in good health, the minority and those over 80 are incapacitated and tend generally to be less aware of services than younger people.
7. *Failure in the supply of services*
People do ask for help and fail to receive it. One study by Scammells [17] examined 150 recipients of health and welfare services. Forty of 150 described how services were demanded but failed to respond effectively. There were 34 examples of failure caused by shortages of supply and 21 instances of administrative breakdown.
8. *Geographical mobility and literacy problems* are two other reasons why services may not be demanded.

THE FUTURE

A study of older people in the north east of Scotland[18] looked at 500 men and women in Aberdeen city and outlying country areas. This study although 17 years old, comments on the diversity of old age, and highlights the discrepancy between services and needs despite impressive post-war increases in statutory and voluntary services. Reading this study illustrates the advances that have been made in the north east of Scotland in housing, sanitation, and the expansion of domiciliary help, yet its comments on the material advances made in the services for elderly people raise the unanswered question of the quality of life and emotional security.

Another survey *Social Welfare for the Elderly*[19] illustrates some of the problems in planning for the future. The survey was a result of doubt expressed by the Governors of the National Corporation for the Care of Old People as to whether the 10 year plans for 1965 - 1976 were based on the *needs* of the elderly or what local authorities could afford.

Harris[19], recognising that local authorities viewed 'need' differently, collected not only the criteria of need as defined by different authorities but compared also how these criteria were administered and also asked the elderly in these areas for their views. Thirteen areas were studied including three in Scotland (Coatbridge, Buckie and Dundee). The study hoped to measure different levels of need using the different standards in different authorities and also simultaneously measure subjective need.

Home helps

The allocation of home helps to elderly people varied. In one area the least possible amount of help was provided for the shortest time, while in another the policy is to give as much help as necessary to keep the home the way the old person would want it kept. Some home helps only clean rooms the elderly live in, others the whole house if a family is resident. It seems to be policy rather than the needs of the elderly or the availability of home helps which determines this.

On average, estimates show that the home help service would at least have to double to cope with new cases of unmet need, in addition to any increase due to the present recipients' needing more help than they can get. In the area with the least unmet need, the service would still have to be expanded by about 40% while in the area with the most unmet need it would have to be quadrupled.

Housing

There was difficulty in getting reliable data as to the number of local authority dwellings occupied by the elderly, or the proportion of housing allocated to them. Even Sheltered Housing was not necessarily allocated to the elderly frail. Waiting lists tended to be out of date. Many authorities wrote to the applicant each year and if they got no reply crossed them off the waiting list - but of course the elderly may not reply due to reasons of frailty etc.

The resident length in area qualification and the likelihood of being rehoused did not tally well. Registration varied - e.g. as to whether an owner-occupier could be rehoused. In some areas local authority tenants were given priority (and then those living in old houses). Some variation existed in how near the old home the elderly person is rehoused.

A lot of unmet need still exists. Some old people go into residential homes for housing need alone.

Residential homes

Most single widowed ladies 75+ have either been living alone or in boarding houses or lodging houses. Most go into a Home because they cannot look after themselves, a few for reasons of loneliness and a few for financial reasons, but at least one in five go in because of accommodation reasons. Most said they were happy in residential care - only 11% were unhappy, but 10% of old people in their own homes were as unhappy. Harris[19] estimated that only 5% both wanted and could live in their own homes if sufficient places were available. In only three areas was it estimated that a large expansion of Homes was needed.

How is any local authority to plan its services?

The average proportion of elderly people allocated a home help in the 13 areas was 4.8 compared to the national figure of 4.5 and meals on wheels 0.9 compared to 1.1. The survey was a mixture of demand and assessed need (i.e. whether housebound, unable to do jobs etc.). This gives a picture of need for an area, but in individual cases the correlation between need and demand is not high (e.g. an individual may be assessed for a service but not want it). To make a general estimate is difficult; the numbers in need do not correlate exactly with numbers of specific groups e.g. those living alone, the older elderly. To obtain a reasonable estimate a considerable number of these interconnected variables have to be considered.

However before making estimates local authorities should assess if their own policies are being borne out in practice - e.g. if underoccupation is a good enough reason for rehousing does it apply only to local authority tenants or all elderly in an area. Need will not be brought to attention where services are inadequate, e.g. if GPs know there are no home helps they will not refer. Demand as a basis is just as likely to underestimate need than open the flood gates. People think a service does not apply to them or do not like to beg, etc. To counteract this misconception publicity is required.

Plank[20] reviews research and provides an overview of the position of elderly people in society with particular reference to the contribution of statutory personal social services and of social work. In looking at need he finds that there is a large number of elderly people with mental health problems and dementia who are receiving no medical or social support either for themselves or those who are looking after them at home. From his review of the research literature he concludes that mental health is only one problem for the elderly; he cites the example of hearing impairment which remain either unrecognised or undetected. The reasons for failure to pick up problems are firstly an undermanned and undertrained health service, secondly the inability to identify and alleviate deterioration in the elderly person by those most in contact, and third the societal belief that physical and mental ill health are inevitable in old age. Plank voices his fear that those old people who do expose their problems in the present situation to the statutory services may be shortening their independence and risking premature institutionalisation. He notes that despite a considerable expansion of services we have still been unable to match services with need, due not only to inadequate resources, but also the failure to respond flexibly to the needs of the elderly. He argues that the needs of the elderly are both complex and extensive in nature and practical help in itself is insufficient. Applications for residential placements are often treated by social workers as administrative procedures rather than key life events, and Plank feels a more sophisticated response to these applications is required by agencies, so that people are not admitted to an old people's home simply because a vacancy exists. He suggests there is an inadequate commitment of social work time to investigate and ameliorate the deteriorating situation which precipitate the decision to request residential care. He recognises that some requests for simple practical help are dealt with by social workers through a short term response, and wonders whether this simple request might not be an indication of an imminent deterioration which in the long term might lead to residential care and might have been prevented by the social worker assessing the overall rather than the presenting needs of the elderly person.

Plank asserts that social work with the elderly is one of the greatest challenges to the social work profession. He recognises that most social work with the elderly is currently being undertaken by untrained social workers while qualified social workers see working with the elderly as unattractive and lacking in challenge. He questions this view stating that the decision to admit to care, the management of the preadmission crisis and preparation for admission demands a high level of social work skill.

Plank also asserts that some people are admitted to residential care because their needs cannot be met in the community out of the social services working hours. It would be too expensive to pay staff to work anti-social hours and there has been inadequate investment in the production of alarm systems or recruiting helping networks of neighbours and helpers. In spelling out the implications for the future, Plank sees the need for a system of care that prolongs elderly people's independence and reduces deterioration. He sees the field social worker as the co-ordinator of social service and health provision, and as a case manager to be responsible for the greater allocation of qualified social work time to the elderly and their families. He envisages the elderly themselves developing a self help role. He also advocates need for a redefined role for residential and day care centres as joint social and health service provisions offering medical help assessment and rehabilitation for the elderly living in their own homes. In those cases where elderly people were admitted to Homes the case would not be closed and the social worker would remain responsible.

CONCLUSION

In this paper an attempt has been made to highlight key factors and findings from a few selected research reports. The international research stressed the problems of elderly people in modern industrial society including our own. The cross-cultural study illustrated how varied are the needs and services for the elderly in Europe, dependent again on culture and ideology. The American research illustrated the experience of being old and stereotyped as such. Retirement, poverty and loneliness were then examined as being inevitable results of political policies rather than pathological symptoms of being old. The United Kingdom studies illustrate the difficulty of discovering the needs of the elderly let alone providing services for unmet needs. The Task Force study suggested eight major factors that reflect difficulties experienced by elderly people in expressing their needs. The survey on local authorities examined the way local authorities defined need of the elderly in terms of local policies, how much they could afford and the complex relationship between supply and demand, questioning whether the elderly would be referred for services that were not supplied, thus obscuring real need.

Plank reviews research on the elderly; he was concerned that failure of the social worker to make an early assessment might be a factor in forcing admission to care, and that work with the elderly did not receive the commitment from trained and experienced social workers it needed. Finally his implications for future coordinated care were summarised.

In preparing this paper gaps in research have been noted and are listed below.

Gaps in research

1. The need for longitudinal studies to plot the 'careers' of elderly people indicating warning signs of predictive significance for service provision.
2. The relationship between the provison of services and consumer satisfaction is another factor that needs more research.
3. Investigation into the feasibility of involving the elderly in planning services so that it is work *with* the elderly rather than possible unwanted or irrelevant services delivered *to* the elderly.
4. Research into the use of Section 47 of the National Assistance Act 1948 invoked in those cases where the elderly person's needs cannot be met by available community services, but where the person refuses to leave their home voluntarily. The social worker must decide to either leave the person 'to die at home' or arrange compulsory removal to a residential home. Official reports have tended to be critical of social work decision making and the deficiencies in service provision. Research is required to examine the effectiveness of Section47, or the the need for amendment.
5. Research is required into the 'quality' of life for the elderly person living with their children and the implications for the family's life.

Acknowledgement

I wish to acknowledge and thank Elizabeth Reinach for all the help she has given in the preparation of this paper.

REFERENCES

1. DHSS. *Growing Older.* HMSO, Cmnd 8173.
2. Cargill, D.O. & Holmes, L.D. *Ageing & Modernisation*, New York Appleton Century, 1972, p.25 - 27.
3. Amann, A.(Ed.) *Open Care for the Elderly in Seven European Countries: a Pilot Study in the Possibilities & Limits of Care*, Pergamon Press, 1980.
4. *The Relationship between Social Security and Social Services.* Reports of the United Nations, 1963 & 1970 (same title).
5. Streib, G.F. 'Family Patterns' in *Retirement Journal of Social Issues* 24, 1958, pp 46-60.
6. Townsend, P. & Tunstall, S. 'Isolation, Desolation & Loneliness' in Shanas, E. & Townsend, P. (Eds.) *Old People in Three Industrial Societies*, 1968, pp 258 - 287.
7. Harris, L. & Associates, *The Myth & Reality of Ageing in America.* Washington D.C. The National Council on the Ageing Inc., 1975.
8. Hendricks, J. & Hendricks, C.D. *Ageing in Mass Society*, Cambridge, Mass., Windthrop, 1975.
9. Isaacs, B. 'Standing Old People on their Heads'. *Community Health* No. 6, 1974, p. 142.
10. Brearley, P. 'Welfare Goals' in Dickson, N. (Ed.) *Living in the 80s, What prospects for the elderly?* Age Concern, England, 1980.
11. Abrams, M. *Beyond Three Score & Ten.* Age Concern, England, 1978.
12. Palmore, E. 'Compulsory versus flexible retirement issues and facts' in *The Gerontologist*, 124, 1972, pp343-8.
13. Townsend, P. *The Failure to House Britain's Aged.* Help the Aged, 1977.
14. Social Survey Division Office of Population Censuses and Surveys. *General Household Survey.* Introductory report, London, HMSO, 1973.
15. Gruer, R. *Needs of the Elderly in the Scottish Borders.* Scottish Home and Health Department, 1975.
16. Chapman, P. *Unmet Need and the Delivery of Care.* Occasional Papers on Social Administration, Willmer Bros. Birkenhead, 1979.
17. Scammells, B. *The Administration of Health & Welfare Services.* Manchester University Press, 1971, p. 100.
18. Richardson, I.M. *Age & Need: a study of Older People in North East Scotland.* Edinburgh, Livingstone, 1964.
19. Harris, A.I. *Social Welfare for the Elderly*, Government Social Survey, London, HMSO, 1968.
20. Plank, D. *What Next for Elderly People?* an overvi ew of service provision and research concerning Elderly Mentally Infirm People. MIND, 1979.

FURTHER READING

I have chosen two books out of a number which significantly advance our knowledge regarding provision for elderly persons.

Goldberg, E.M. & Connelly, N.
The Effectiveness of Social Care for the Elderly: an Overview of Recent and Current Evaluative Research. Heinemann, London, 1982.

Coming from the Policy Studies Institute, this book starts with what evaluation is, why and how it is carried out. It then addresses itself to an evaluation of Care in the Community in terms of Domiciliary Care, Social Work, Day

Care Services and Voluntary Action. Finally it evaluates special accommodation in terms of Assisted Lodgings and Sheltered Housing and Residential Care.

The major findings of this book reflect implications for policy for the tasks of home help organisers who were not always able to use their home helps in the best way possible either with regard to matching or geographical allocation. Many people who received meals on wheels would have preferred help with shopping, and residents in homes for elderly people wanted to influence their environment in terms of opening windows and controlling radiators.

Studies with experimental outcomes are examined which looked at different ways of providing services other than those currently being provided. Although small in scale they are of significance. The book also describes small controlled experiments in residential settings aimed at enhancing the quality of life and engagement levels with elderly people. Another group of experiments examine life styles: group living, mutual help and preservation of self care.

Methods and tools of investigation are examined with regard to monitoring of services, attempts are described to measure 'life satisfaction' and 'morale' as well as measures of disability and dependency. The currency of assessments are discussed in terms of whether they are needs based, or based on services available and whether they are needed yet unrequested or overprovided. This book goes a long way in presenting research findings for policy makers and fills in some gaps previously identified. This book is a source of most significant research findings.

Kayser-Jones, J.K.
Old, Alone, and Neglected. Care of the Aged in Scotland and the United States. University of California Press, California, 1981.

This book contrasts 'Scottsdale', an N.H.S. hospital for 96 chronically ill patients over 65 years of age in Scotland, with 'Pacific Manor' a unit for 95 patients in the United States. At the time of writing, 1981, about a million elderly Americans lived in residential nursing homes which were, according to Kayser-Jones, often impersonal, below standard and tended to infantilisation, depersonalisation, dehumanisation and victimisation. These homes were also privately owned and motivated to make financial profits.

In contrast the Scottish N.H.S. institution studied was found to be pleasant, with high standards, the elderly being treated as individuals with useful work and social experiences even though located in old buildings. Kayser-Jones concludes that the structure of the health care system in Scotland promotes care of high quality while in the United States the system of privatised health care leads to stigmatisation and pauperisation of the elderly.

This book is particularly pertinent at a time when the growth of private facilities for the elderly has mushroomed in Britain without any corresponding attention to standards of care or public accountability as currently exists in N.H.S. hospitals and local authority homes for elderly persons.

Relevant Statistics

David Goda

INTRODUCTION

'The man in the street regards statistical data with a fair amount of suspicion; and not without good reason. Statistics are sometimes used with gross dishonesty to present, for political purposes, a deliberately misleading picture of social or economic reality. More often, statistical data have placed upon them a greater weight of interpretation than they can really support, or have inappropriate or irrelevant conclusions drawn from them. These latter misuses do not necessarily stem from any intention to defraud or confuse, but generally reflect a lack of thoughtful awareness of the nature of the data in question and of the ways in which they are constructed. It would be a mistake however to conclude that the honest man would do well to wash his hands of statistics. If figures can mislead, by design or by accident, so too - and no less powerfully - can words, or indeed any means of human communication. But it is incumbent on the consumer to use information thoughtfully and critically, with a due sense of its limitations and possible biases.' (Martin, 1976)

That paragraph opened a discussion of statistical patterns in the children's hearings system, but is equally relevant to this brief examination of the official statistical information available concerning elderly people in Scotland and the services available to them.

The biggest limitation and possible bias stems from the lack of an agreed definition of the word 'elderly'. In part, this follows from the fact that age is not itself a handicap, an illness or a disability. Problems and chronological age tend to be confused and 'the elderly' becomes a shorthand for a range of different subgroups - people of pensionable age, retired people, people in poor physical or mental health, and so on. The various statistical systems reflect this confusion, making it very difficult to obtain a clear view of the pattern of services used by older people.

One example suffices here. Various social work returns either leave the term 'elderly' undefined or (following the Chronically Sick and Disabled Persons Acts) include everybody over 65. Thus for example a 64 year old blind person receiving home care services will be recorded as 'physically handicapped'; the next year he will only be 'age 65-74'. It would seem that the handicap or problem is regarded as relevant only for the youngest 9% of recipients.

An important characteristic of services for the elderly is that provision is made by a variety of agencies, operating in separate systems, at different levels of administration, responsible for different geographical areas. In Scotland, these include the (Great Britain) Department of Health & Social Security, the area health boards, the regional social work departments, the district authorities (providing, particularly, sheltered housing but also in some areas social facilities), voluntary social work agencies and housing associations. In general we know little about the ways in which the provision of one service influences demand for or provision of another. The relationships obviously depend not only upon need but also for example upon criteria for access to each service, which in turn depend upon demand and provision. We do know that individuals may use several services at the same or different times. For example a resident in sheltered housing may receive home help and meals on wheels, or attend a lunch club, and be a hospital out-patient, but may become more frail and require admission to a home for the elderly.

There has been little quantitative research into the patterns of service in different areas and the ways in which services can and do interact. Studies have generally been restricted to a limited range of services, or to people in a particular kind of accommodation, or to one area. Most, too, have been so limited in time that there has been scarcely any analysis of the different services used by the same individual over a period. Cumming (1968) examined the patterns of service contacts over time, but her work (in the United States) was not especially directed to services for the elderly.

The available statistical information is, moreover, almost wholly service-based. This is exemplified by the treatment of the elderly in successive issues of 'Social Trends'. The 1973 volume carried a special article on 'The Elderly'; its author, D.C.L. Wroe, explicitly admitted (p.33) 'The present paper does not claim to have fully exploited the available information.' Subsequent issues have included a short chapter with the same title, but the commentary and tables have all been service-based, except for part of one table in the 1979 edition, based on the 1971 census. The first substantial attempt to collate information from the various agencies providing services for the elderly in Scotland has, we believe, been my own recent work for Social Work Services Group. Until final results are available, my claims for this paper are no stronger than Mr. Wroe's, eight years ago.

A further problem is that statistics are compiled for different services at different dates. Various patient/case/client and service statistics used in this paper relate to the position at, or the year ending, 31 December 1979 and 31 March 1980. Some staffing statistics are compiled as at 30 September each year. As the paper was being prepared, only a few preliminary analyses were available from the census of population held in April 1981, and none by age or by household composition. Although estimates and projections of populations are published annually by the General Register Office for Scotland, the decennial census is the only source of reliable national data on the circumstances in which elderly people live. Parts of the next section had therefore to be based on data more than ten years old.

Finally in this introductory section, it should be made clear that the paper has attempted to collate demographic data and official national statistics on the provision of housing, health and social work services. No mention is made of the literature on need for services, and questions of income and wealth are excluded.

DEMOGRAPHIC TRENDS

Table 1 and figure 1 show the total population of Scotland, and the numbers aged over 65, over 75 and over 85, at each census from 1851 to 1971; mid-year estimates for 1939 and 1979; and projections from 1979 to 1989, 1999, 2009 and 2019. The projections are not intended to be precise estimates of what the population will be; rather, they are projections of what it would be on certain hypotheses about the trends of future births, deaths and migration. In figure 1, the vertical scale is logarithmic and each age group is shown as a percentage of its numbers in 1931, the middle point of the series.

Over the 120 years to 1971, the total population of Scotland increased by 81%, from under 3 million to over 5 million. During the following 48 years, from 1971 to the limit of the available projections, it is likely to fall back by 5% to just under 5 million. Over the whole period of 168 years from 1851 to 2019, by contrast, the number of people aged over 65 will have increased more than five-fold, those over 75 by 6½ times, and those over 85 by 10½ times - from fewer than 7,000 to more than 70,000.

TABLE 1

THE ELDERLY POPULATION OF SCOTLAND 1851 - 2019 [*Thousands*]

Date	Persons all ages (2)	Age last birthday (1) 65 +	75 +	85 +
1851 Census	2,888.7	137.8	44.9	6.9
1861 Census	3,062.3	149.2	48.3	6.9
1871 Census	3,360.0	174.0	52.0	7.3
1881 Census	3,735.6	186.0	57.9	7.2
1891 Census	4,025.6	203.1	63.2	8.6
1901 Census	4,472.1	216.5	65.5	8.4
1911 Census	4,760.9	257.4	72.4	9.3
1921 Census	4,882.5	291.9	85.0	10.6
1931 Census	⌈4,843.0	353.2	98.3	11.5
1939 Estimate (3)	5,006.7	...	...	...
1951 Census	⌊5,096.4	506.9	163.4	19.8
1961 Census	5,179.3	548.9	190.5	27.2
1971 Census	5,229.0	644.5	217.9	37.2
1979 Estimate	5,167.0	717.8	259.9	42.9
1989 Projected	5,153.0	726.6	303.8	57.8
1999 Projected	5,144.0	706.3	302.9	68.8
2009 Projected	5,025.0	685.3	298.0	71.7
2019 Projected	4,965.0	742.0	296.0	72.7

Moreover, the population aged 65 and over will reach a temporary peak in 1988, then falling to reflect the low birth-rate of the 1930s and early 40s, before climbing again 65 years after the 'post-war bulge'. The number of very elderly people, those aged over 85, will continue to increase well into the next century. The number aged over 85 per 10,000 total population, which fell from 24 in 1851 to 19 in 1901, has since then steadily increased, reaching 83 in 1979, and is projected to continue increasing to 146 in 2019. Figure 2 seeks to throw some light on these changing patterns by graphing the expectations of life for men and women at selected ages, as calculated from records of deaths during various periods from 1861-70 until 1978. Over a little more than a century, the expectations of life at birth has increased for males from 40 to 68 years, and for females from 44 to 74 years - an increase of 69% in each case. For men who have reached the age of 65, by contrast, the further expectation of life has increased by only 9%, from 10.8 to 11.8 years. For females, the increase beyond age 65 is

FIGURE 1
THE ELDERLY POPULATION OF SCOTLAND, 1851 - 2019

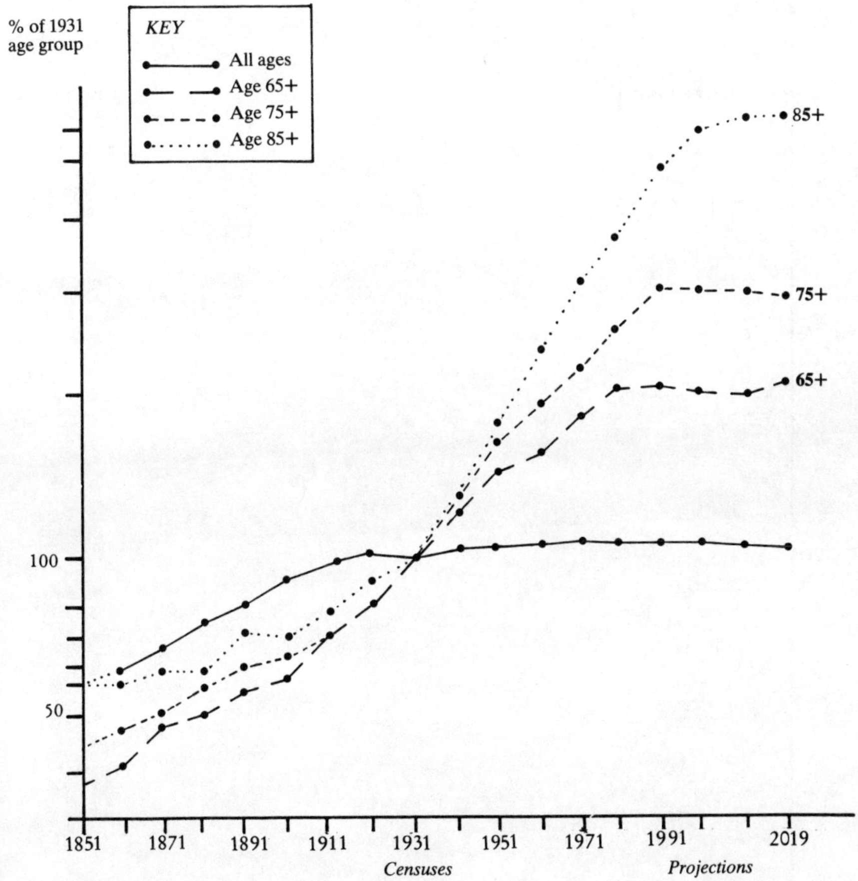

34%, from 11.6 years to 15.6 years. In essence, the major changes have been the increased survival of small children, particularly during the first year of life, and of what we now regard as young adults, in their 20s and 30s. A century ago, the expectation of life at birth was around 45 years; it was fairly rare to reach the age of 60, but many of those who did so were fit enough to survive several more years. Now it is normal to survive at least until 60, but those who do so have little greater expectation of further survival than had their ancestors.

FIGURE 2
EXPECTATION OF LIFE IN SCOTLAND, 1861 - 1978

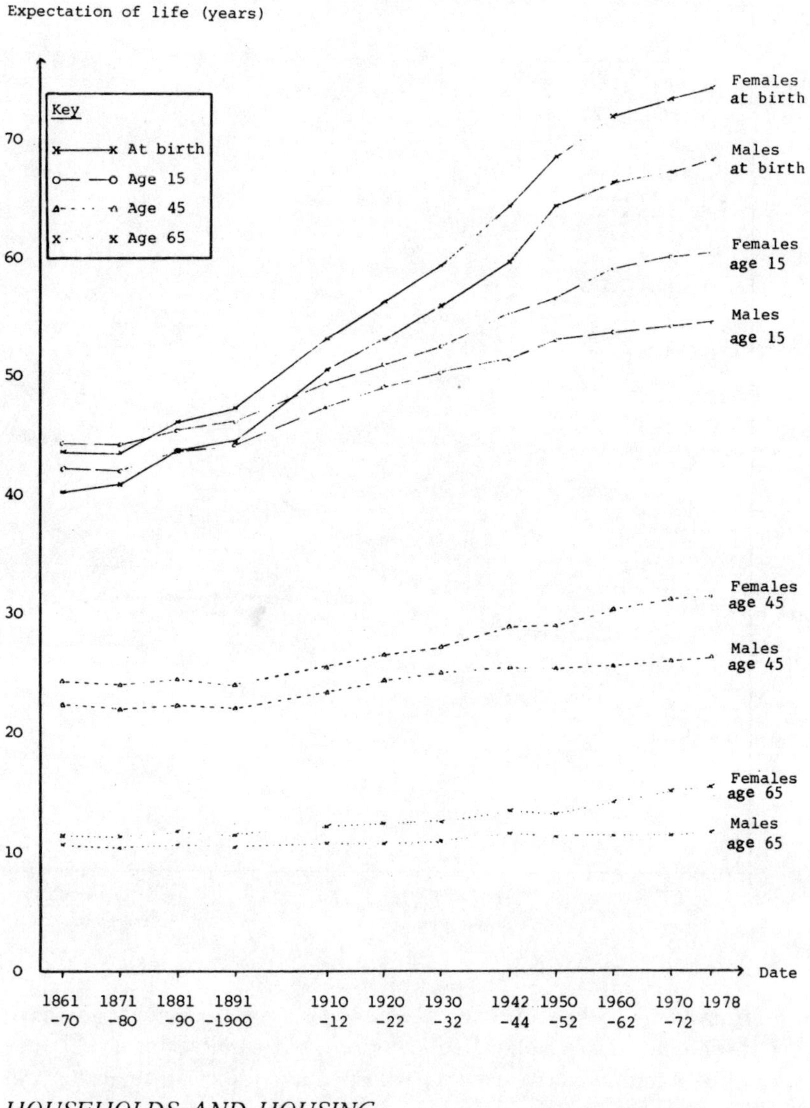

HOUSEHOLDS AND HOUSING

Some of the relevant information from the population and household composition analyses of the 1971 census is presented in tables 2A and 2B. The census definition of a household may be misleading in some relevant

TABLE 2A
CENSUS 1971 SCOTLAND: PERSONS OF PENSIONABLE AGE BY PLACE OF ENUMERATION [*Thousands*]

Place of enumeration	Males 65 +	Females 60 +	Total persons
Persons in private households - total	229.4	526.7	756.1
- in one-person households	33.9	170.0	203.9
- in two-person households	126.4	227.0	353.4
- in other households	69.1	129.7	198.7
Persons not in private households - total	15.4	32.3	47.7
- in hospitals etc.	8.2	18.7	26.9
- in homes for the old and the disabled	3.8	8.4	12.2
- in hotels and boarding houses	1.7	3.0	4.7
- in other establishments and elsewhere (1)	1.6	2.3	3.8
Total persons over pensionable age	244.8	559.0	803.7

TABLE 2B
CENSUS 1971 SCOTLAND: PERSONS OF PENSIONABLE AGE IN PRIVATE HOUSEHOLDS [*Thousands*]

Household type (1)	Males 65 +	Females 60 +	Total persons	Persons 75 +	
				Males	Females
One person	33.8	176.1	209.9	12.4	55.2
Married couple, no others	112.8	145.9	258.7	25.1	15.2
Married couple with others (2)	53.3	79.6	133.0	14.4	19.0
Lone parent (3)	11.7	55.6	67.2	5.6	19.6
Other household types	21.2	72.6	93.8	6.6	21.5
Total persons over pensionable age in private households	232.7	529.8	762.5	64.2	130.6

circumstances and it is for example impossible from the published tables to deduce the number of households comprising elderly siblings. It is nevertheless clear that nearly 95% of those beyond the normal retirement ages were living in private households, and almost 90% even of those over 75. For people aged between 60/65 and 74, the largest group comprised married couples living in two person households, followed by unmarried or widowed women living alone. Among those over 75, women living alone formed the largest group.

Since many of the categories used in earlier censuses were different, few comparisons are possible. One simple comparison can however be made between 1961 and 1971, and the trend is believed to have continued. The total number of people over pensionable age increased over the decade by 22% but the numbers living alone almost doubled; the increase was broadly similar for each sex and each age band[1].

The census also collects valuable information on household tenure, number of rooms and so on. Between censuses, much information about households and housing is obtained by various surveys, but none has a sufficient sample of elderly people throughout Scotland to be relevant to this paper. The Scottish Development Department does however collect information on sheltered and amenity housing, which is summarised in table 3. The figures refer to provision, not utilisation, but the overwhel-

TABLE 3
SHELTERED AND AMENITY HOUSING, 31:3:80

	Local authority	Housing association (1) (2)
Sheltered dwellings	6,335	1,971
(No. of bedspaces)	10,839	(2,760)
Amenity dwellings	3,795	143
Sheltered wheelchair dwellings	173	38

ming majority of the dwellings concerned are occupied by old people. From time to time, the figures have been amended as particular dwellings move into and out of changing definitions of sheltered and amenity housing. The total number of old people living in sheltered or amenity dwellings provided by local authorities and by housing associations may be estimated at around 20,000. This represents about 2.8% of all those aged 65 and over, rather fewer than are hospital in-patients at any given date but half as many again as are residents in homes for the elderly.

HOSPITAL IN-PATIENT AND HOME RESIDENTS

Of all hospital in-patient bed days in 1979, excluding psychiatric and maternity, 63% were occupied by patients aged over 65, indeed 30% by women over 75, who comprised only 3.4% of the general population[2]. Since relatively little information is available about hospital patients by

TABLE 4A
HOSPITAL IN-PATIENTS, SELECTED SPECIALTIES,
1:4:79 - 31:3:80(1)

Specialty	Average available staffed beds	Average occupied beds	Discharges and deaths
Geriatric assessment	2,475	2,289	12,638
Geriatric long stay	7,805	7,440	7,550
Psychogeriatric	2,523	2,396	2,009
GP acute and long stay	1,132	959	11,720
General medicine	4,508	3,817	107,764
Orthopaedic surgery	2,759	2,130	47,193
Mental illness	14,467	12,797	22,948
Total all specialties	59,856	50,069	733,379

age, table 4A gives some statistics for the specialties most used by the elderly. Geriatric and psychogeriatric beds, so-called, comprise just over a fifth of all the hospital beds in Scotland, although these include some occupied by younger chronically sick patients. But elderly patients also occupy a large proportion of the beds in several other specialties, notably general medicine, orthopaedic surgery and mental illness, and general practitioner acute and long stay beds. Some health boards have no explicitly psychogeriatric beds, treating such patients in the general psychiatric wards.

Further information is available from the Scottish Hospital In-patient Statistics. The main system, which excludes hospitals and units for mental illness, mental deficiency and maternity, is based upon a return for each discharge (including deaths, but also transfers from one specialty to another in the same hospital). Of the discharges recorded in this system in 1979, 29% involved patients aged over 65 and 14% patients over 75[3]. Before discharge, however, female patients over the age of 75 spent on average nearly seven times as long in the hospital as those under 65; for women between 65 and 74 the corresponding ratio was 3:1[4]. The difference was less for males, with ratios of 3½:1 (75+) and 2¼:1 (65-74).

Table 4B shows 13 diagnostic groups which together accounted for 85% of the bed days occupied by patients over 65. Most bed days were necessitated by cerebrovascular disease (stroke), followed by pneumonia and heart diseases. The total of 5.6 million bed days for patients over 65

TABLE 4B
HOSPITAL IN-PATIENT BED DAYS, SELECTED DIAGNOSES, 1979 [Thousands] (1)

Diagnostic group	Males 65 - 74	Males 75 +	Females 65 - 74	Females 75 +	Grand total All ages
Malignant neoplasms	109.4	82.4	102.7	111.8	652.7
Mental disorders	16.1	22.8	28.3	161.7	286.3
Diseases of central nervous system	52.9	45.7	78.6	109.4	562.2
Heart diseases	95.0	117.6	113.2	327.7	871.6
Cerebrovascular disease	134.6	120.0	178.6	491.6	1,056.5
Other diseases of circulatory system	45.3	44.2	52.7	132.8	379.2
Pneumonia	58.3	121.4	91.2	439.9	773.8
Other diseases of respiratory system	57.1	69.2	36.1	79.2	417.9
Diseases of digestive system	48.6	41.6	56.4	86.0	542.2
Rheumatoid arthritis, osteoarthritis and allied conditions	18.0	17.1	63.5	99.9	273.2
"Other and ill-defined conditions"	37.1	46.4	49.5	129.3	464.3
Fracture of neck of femur	8.4	18.3	28.6	140.3	223.0
Other fractures, dislocations and sprains	13.3	13.1	30.8	80.3	288.9
Total all diagnoses	845.1	907.2	1,090.4	2,758.3	8,931.0

meant that on average elderly patients occupied 15,350 beds at any time, just over 10,000 of these patients being over 75. In addition, the residents at 31 December 1979 of mental hospitals, psychiatric units and mental handicap hospitals included 3,964 patients aged 65-74 and 5,584 over 75[5]. On average, therefore, patients in all types of hospital represented at any time 2% of the general population aged between 65 and 74, and 6% of those over 75; the corresponding figure for those under 65 - including maternity[6] - was 0.7%.

Table 5 gives some of the available statistics for the residential homes for the elderly provided by local authorities, or managed by voluntary agencies or privately and registered with social work departments. The total number of occupants aged 65 and over on 31 March 1980 was 12,825; thus these homes accommodated ½% of the population aged 65-74, 2½% of those 75-84 and 11% of everybody over 85 years old. Of residents aged 65 and over, 36% were physically handicapped, 5% mentally handi-

TABLE 5
HOMES FOR THE ELDERLY, 31:3:80

	Local authority	Registered
No. of homes	247	175
Bed complement	9,348	5,084
Occupants - total	8,788	4,642
- under 65	425	180
- 65-74	1,631	691
- 75-84	3,763	1,951
- 85 +	2,969	1,820
Discharges and deaths - total	4,188	1,435

capped and 4% mentally ill; 4% were recorded as chairbound or bedfast, 10% regularly incontinent and 16% mentally confused[7].

DOMICILIARY HEALTH AND SOCIAL WORK SERVICES

TABLE 6
DOMICILIARY HEALTH SERVICES, 1979

	All ages	65 - 74	75 +
Health visiting -			
patients	532,000	39,300	57,000
visits	2,078,100	145,000	267,100
mean visits/patient	3.9	3.7	4.7
Home nursing -			
patients	156,700	36,400	64,100
visits	4,217,000	1,097,400	2,278,400
mean visits/patient	26.9	30.1	35.5

Table 6 provides some summary statistics for the health visiting and home nursing services in 1979. The former primarily assists young families, but 22% of the population aged over 75 (and therefore around 24% of those not in institutional accommodation) were seen by a health visitor at least once during the year[8]. The home nursing service, by contrast, is largely a service for the elderly, patients over 65 comprising 64% of the caseload and 80% of visits. Almost 25% of the population aged 75 and over were visited during the year by a district nurse; 8% of those aged 65-74 were also visited. Unfortunately, no information is available on the extent to which some elderly people are visited during the year by both a health visitor and a district nurse, and indeed receive one or more social work services too.

TABLE 7
DOMICILIARY SOCIAL WORK SERVICES, 1:4:79 - 31:3:80

	All ages	65 +
Home help service -		
cases open at 31 March	60,700	55,100
cases closed during year	24,800	21,100
Meals-on-wheels -		
meals served in year	1,863,000	...
recipients at 31 March	14,900	...

Table 7 summarises the main domiciliary services provided to the elderly by the social work departments. In addition, at least 11,000 elderly people were 'allocated' to social workers or community occupational therapists [9]. As at 31 March 1980, 8% of people over 65 were receiving home help service; the average client received about 6 hours' service per week[10]. Information on the relative proportions under and over 75 years old is unfortunately incomplete, but just over two-thirds of recipients were over 75 in those areas for which the data are available[11]. The figures imply that some 22% of those over 75 living in private households received home help service at some time during the year. The proportion may indeed be higher: when for example the service is provided for an elderly couple, it is usually allocated in the statistical records to the wife alone.

No information is available about the ages of meals on wheels recipients, but it is believed that the overwhelming majority are elderly. In many areas, this service is provided for the social work department on an agency basis by a voluntary organisation, often the Women's Royal Voluntary Service. Over half the recipients receive two meals per week, almost all the remainder three, four or five[12].

Little information is available about a number of other services for the elderly, including day hospitals, clubs and day centres. More than 600 luncheon clubs provided by or in contact with the social work departments serve over 2½ million meals annually[13]. In addition, some 60 social clubs and day centres for the elderly provide in total 3,700 places[14] in a form of provision which has grown rapidly in recent years. The numbers of individual elderly people using these various services is unknown.

LOCAL VARIATIONS

This paper has briefly examined some aspects of Scottish demography and of the services used by the elderly. No consideration has been given to the large variations which exist between districts within Scotland. These are the subject of current research and a few examples must suffice here. Of every 1,000 people in Scotland, 138 are over 65. Among the 34 health districts, the figure ranges from 90 in West Lothian to 193 in the Western Isles[15]. Similarly, 8 of every 1,000 in Scotland are over 85, only 4 in Monklands/Cumbernauld but 12 in Argyll & Bute and in Angus. During 1979, health visitors saw (once at least) 210 of every 1,000 people over 75 in Scotland. Statistics are not available for every health district, but among the 15 health board areas the rate ranged from 55 in Orkney and 75 in Argyll & Clyde to 510 in Grampian[16]. There was only a slight tendency for each patient to be visited more often in areas where fewer of the population were patients; nor did the district nurses compensate, indeed they tended to visit more people over 75 where the health visitors did likewise[17].

NOTES TO TABLES

General

Where, in certain tables, figures have been rounded, slight differences may be found between the sums of constituent entries and the total shown. The symbol '...' means not available.

Table 1 and Figure 1

(1) The numbers 65 + include those 75 + and the numbers 75 + include those 85 + .

(2) The census figures are the populations enumerated in Scotland; the estimates are for the home population at mid-year, i.e. the population of all types actually in Scotland; the projections (which are based on the 1979 estimates) relate to the total population, i.e. home population plus members of H.M. Forces or the Merchant Navy of Scottish domicile but, serving overseas, minus members of other countries' forces temporarily stationed in Scotland.

(3) No census was taken in 1941.

Sources: Census 1971 Scotland, Population Tables, tables 1 and 13. Annual Estimates of the Population of Scotland 1979. Population Projections Microfiche 1979-2019 (OPCS series PP2, No. 11).

Table 2A

(1) Includes campers, vagrants and certain of those enumerated in caravans.

Source: Census 1971 Scotland, Population Tables, tables 36 and 37.

Table 2B

(1) The household composition tables were based on the 'de jure' or 'usually resident' population. In particular, they included household members absent from their usual address on census night. Thus the totals are larger than those in table 2A, based on the place of enumeration.

(2) Includes both elderly couples with their never-married child(ren) - who may themselves be elderly - and younger couples with for example a widowed parent.

(3) A mother or father together with his or her never-married child(ren), with or without others.

Source: Census 1971 Scotland, Household Composition Tables (100%), table 4.

Figure 2

Source: Annual Report of the Registrar General for Scotland 1978, table J1.1.

Table 3

(1) Includes provision by new town development corporations.

(2) Includes provision in two districts by the Scottish Special Housing Association.

(3) No information is available for two districts.

Source: Information supplied by Scottish Development Department.
N.B. The figures in the first edition were incorrect.

Table 4A

(1) Beds in joint user and contractual hospitals are included in the data.

Sources: Hospital Bed Resources, year ended 31 March, 1980. Hospital Utilisation Statistics, year ending 31 March, 1980, tables A, X and Y.

Table 4B

(1) Excluding hospitals and units for mental illness, mental deficiency and maternity.

Source: Scottish Hospital In-patient Statistics 1979, table 2.

Table 5

Sources: Social Work Services Group Statistical Bulletin RA3/1981, table 1. Information supplied by Social Work Services Group.

Table 6

Source: Scottish Health Statistics 1979, tables 8.12 and 8.13.

Table 7

Sources: Social Work Services Group Statistical Bulletin HD3/1981, tables 3 and 4. Information supplied by Social Work Services Group.

REFERENCES

Cumming, E. (1968) *Systems of Social Regulation,* Atherton Press.
Martin, F.M. (1976) Children and the hearings: some statistical patterns. In Martin, F.M. and Murray, K. *Children's Hearings,* Scottish Academic Press.

NOTES ON THE TEXT

1. Census 1961 Scotland, Household Composition Tables, table 11.
2. Scottish Hospital In-patient Statistics 1979, table 2.
3. Ibid.
4. Ibid.
5. Scottish Mental Hospital In-patient Statistics 1979, table 10.
6. Information supplied by Information Services Division, Common Services Agency for the Scottish Health Service.
7. Social Work Services Statistical Bulletin RA3/1981, table 13. The categories overlap: for example 2% of residents (including those under 65) were both physically and mentally handicapped - see table 15.
8. The mean of 4.7 visits per patient over 75 should not be interpreted as an average of one visit every eleven weeks, since often several visits will be made during a period of crisis.
9. Social Work Services Group Statistical Bulletin C3/1981, tables 1, 12 and 16. In Scotland excluding the Strathclyde Region, at 31 March 1980, there were 12,479 allocated clients over retirement age (60/65) and 7,550 for whom 'elderly and infirm' was recorded as a reason (perhaps one of several) for contact with the social work department. In Strathclyde, 4,061 clients were recorded as 'elderly and infirm' but the figures are not comparable since only one reason for contact was recorded. In many instances physical handicap was recorded as the main reason for contact with elderly people, particularly by occupational therapists (ibid., p.3).
10. Social Work Services Group Statistical Bulletin HD3/1981, table 1. Little information is available nationally about patterns of service. The average of 6 hours per week undoubtedly hides a wide range for individual recipients, from one or two hours, once a week, to a very intensive service of several hours each day; 6 hours per week may be 3 hours on each of two weekdays, or one hour daily from Monday to Saturday.
11. Social Work Services Group Statistical Bulletin HD3/1981, table 3 and information supplied by Social Work Services Group.
12. Social Work Services Group Statistical Bulletin HD3/1981, table 4.
13. Ibid., table 5.
14. Ibid., table 18 and information supplied by Social Work Services Group. These statistics are particularly unreliable: services are not necessarily known to the local social work department and recording by the departments is sometimes incomplete.
15. Annual Estimates of the Population of Scotland 1979 and information supplied by the General Register Office for Scotland.
16. Scottish Health Statistics 1979, table 8.12.
17. Ibid., table 8.13.

Lifestyles of the Elderly

Mark Abrams

If we define the elderly as all the men and women in the U.K. now aged 65 or more then we are discussing the behaviour of some 8¼ million people and a constituency where a span of 35 years separates the youngest from the oldest. The life histories of the oldest half-million (i.e. those over 85 years of age) stretch back to a late nineteenth century landscape that included ubiquitous and gargantuan workhouses that housed 10% of all elderly people and provided outdoor relief for another 20%; it was a time when at the turn of the century the total electorate was barely 7 million, the aggregate membership of all trade unions was less than 2 million; there were a million unemployed, but all were citizens of an empire on which 'the sun never set'. In their later years they lived through the Boer War, the Great War, the Second World War, the Great Depression of the 1930's, and then in late middle age they witnessed the launch of Beveridge's Welfare State and began to taste its benefits.

The life history of the youngest half million of today's elderly (i.e. those aged 65) has developed against a background that was showing signs of change. By the time they started school at the age of 5 in 1922 a Conservative Government was about to be replaced by the country's first Labour Government (admittedly briefly and without a majority in the House of Commons); an Education Act had opened up secondary education for a small minority of working class children; death rates among the young from measles, scarlet fever and whooping cough were falling sharply; some women had been given the vote and the total electorate had increased to 21 million; between 1901 and 1921 life expectation at birth had increased in England and Wales by 10 years for both males and females. However, when they left school nine years later in 1931 it was to enter a society where housing conditions were so poor that 10% of the population were living at a rate of more than 2 persons per room (i.e. a typical '2 up and 2 down' was not officially overcrowded if it was occupied by no more than 8 people); and they entered (or failed to enter) an economy where over 20% of insured workers were unemployed. But over the next ten years average material conditions were improving steadily so that between 1931-3 and 1937-8 (the last two complete years of peace before World War II) average real income per head increased by 15%.

When the war ended in 1945 today's youngest half million of elderly people were aged 28 and for the next 25 years and while in the prime of life they were participants in a burst of social, economic and technological change probably unique in the whole of the country's history - full employment and a near doubling of the average standard of living that created mass markets for good housing, refrigerators, television sets, motor cars, holidays, central heating, home ownership, washing machines, telephones, good clothes, credit cards - material assets undreamt of by the oldest half million of today's elderly population when they were young and rarely owned by them even in middle age.

The purpose of these simple sketches is to stress the fact that simply because of difference in historical background we must expect to find a considerable variety of life styles among the elderly; and the variety generated by cohort experience is increased and made more complex by the fact that among the elderly themselves there are differences of income, health, and the availability and use of leisure time; and sometimes these differences within the elderly population are at least as great as those between the elderly and the non-elderly.

INCOME AND LIFE STYLES

At least the second part of the phrase 'the poor get older and the old get poorer' is documented afresh in each issue of the Department of Employment's annual *Family Expenditure Survey*.[1] The most recently published of these describes from a total sample of 6,777 households studied in 1979 the sharp differences in income related to age of the head of household. In that year the gross normal weekly household income where the head was aged 50 and under 65 was £133.76p - a sum more than double that of the £61.92 recorded for households where the head was aged 65 or more. The former group received £108.86 from wages, salaries and self-employment while these three sources provided the elderly household with only £13.38 in gross income. The gap between the gross incomes of the average household in these two age bands was reduced after the payment of direct taxes and deductions for state insurance schemes but even then it realised almost at the level of 2 to 1 - £108.29 for those aged 50 to 64, and £56.06 for those aged 65 or more. Not all disposable income was spent by either group; some was held back for savings etc, and the differences in total household expenditure was still further reduced by differences in family size; households where the head was 65 or more were appreciably smaller. But even when all these adjustments have been made it remains true that weekly expenditure per head was 25% lower among the elderly - £31.17 as compared with £42.01 per head for those aged 50 to 64.

There is, however, a fairly high degree of inequality of income and expenditure among the elderly themselves. For example, in the 1979 *Family Expenditure Survey* there were 1,783 households where the head was aged 65 or more (i.e. 26% of all households) and of these 34% had gross normal weekly incomes of under £35 while 15% had gross weekly incomes of £100 or more. Of course, these two groups differed considerably in the composition of the average household. The typical low income elderly household is small and normally consists of a woman in her mid-seventies living alone. Among the affluent elderly the typical household consists of two or three adults of whom one is a man who is usually still working. The Survey report allows one to take these differences into account by providing separate tables for four groups of retired households: (a) 1 person households mainly dependent on state pensions (i.e. at least three-quarters of the total income of the household is derived from national insurance retirement pensions including supplementary benefits etc.); (b) other 1 person retired households; (c) 1 man and 1 woman retired households mainly dependent on state pensions; (d) other retired households of 1 man and 1 woman. In Table 1, the expenditure on leisure goods and services by groups (a) and (b) are compared; and in Table 2 similar comparisons are made for households consisting of 2 retired people - 1 man and 1 woman (groups (c) and (d)).

These two groups of retired elderly households are identical, or very similar, in size, average age and sex compostion. They differ, of course, in weekly income and expenditure. The total weekly expenditure of the average poor household (group (a)), is little more than half that of the average affluent household (group (b)). The former, somehow, have to manage with £17.48 less. They achieve this in part by making a 35% cut in their expenditure on 'basics' such as housing, food and fuel; but the biggest relative economy is made by a reduction of 64% in their expenditure on leisure goods and services, and this is achieved very largely by

TABLE 1
THE RETIRED 1-PERSON HOUSEHOLD; WEEKLY EXPENDITURE ON LEISURE GOODS AND SERVICES. U.K. 1979

	(a) Mainly dependent on state pensions	(b) Other retired	(a) as % of (b)
Average age	74	73	
Weekly expenditure	£	£	%
Books, newspapers, mags.	.53	.89	60
Gardening goods	.07	.19	37
Alcohol and tobacco	1.05	1.41	75
Cinema admissions	—	.01	—
Photographic and optical goods	.03	.11	27
Hotel, holiday expenses, clubs	.59	2.42	24
Transport and vehicles	.45	2.78	16
Musical instruments, TV etc.	.04	.16	25
Meals out	.31	.61	51
Travel and sports goods etc.	.06	.19	32
Theatres, sporting events	.03	.11	27
Total	3.16	8.88	36
All other expenditure	22.06	33.82	65
Total expenditure	25.22	42.70	59
N =	505	358	
Proportion who are women %	83	76	

spending no more than £1.16 a week in the average week on holidays, club membership fees, public transport and private motoring, cameras etc., travel goods, and admissions to theatres and other entertainments - in short, by cutting themselves off from gregarious activities outside their homes. The affluent retired elderly spend nearly five times as much (£5.61) on these particular leisure goods and services which provide mobility and opportunities for enjoying new places and meeting new people. What the retired elderly 1 person holds on to most tenaciously is her expenditure on newspapers and magazines, alcohol and tobacco - all apparently supports for solitary living in poverty.

Table 2 similarly presents figures of expenditure by the two types of retired households composed of 2 adults - 1 man and 1 woman. In terms of average age, size and age composition of households the two groups are almost identical. They do, of course, differ in total household expenditure; where the household income is mainly derived from state pensions and benefits total expenditure is nearly 30% lower. Again the biggest relative economies made by the poorer household is in expenditure on leisure goods and services where they spend less than half the amount that the average affluent household does. But within the leisure area their economies are not spread evenly; they forego (or have less need for) much expenditure on admission to theatres, cinemas, sporting events, expenditure on restaurant meals, on public transport and private motoring. On the other hand, they spend comparatively liberally on newspapers and magazines, on alcohol and tobacco and, perhaps surprisingly, on holidays; their sustained expenditure on the last of these is almost 60% of that spent by the average affluent retired couple, but that is because the latter apparently spend very little on hotel and holiday expenses and much more on travelling around by car and rail.

The overall picture, however, is much the same as for the 1-person retired individual. The elderly poor couple tends to make do financially by a large relative cut in expenditure on leisure goods and services and they are cuts that primarily involve expenditure by seeking leisure outside the home.

TABLE 2
THE RETIRED 2-PERSON HOUSEHOLD; WEEKLY EXPENDITURE ON LEISURE GOODS AND SERVICES. U.K. 1979

	(a) Mainly dependent on state pensions	(b) Other retired	(a) as % of (b)
Average Age	73	72	
Weekly Expenditure	£	£	%
Books, newspapers, mags.	.90	1.29	70
Gardening goods	.22	.62	36
Alcohol and tobacco	3.03	4.26	71
Cinema admissions	—	.01	—
Photographic and optical goods	.09	.22	41
Hotel, holiday expenses, clubs	1.09	1.85	59
Transport and vehicles	2.29	7.11	32
Musical instruments, TV etc.	.21	.62	34
Meals out	.39	1.17	33
Travel and sports goods etc.	.20	.47	43
Theatres, sporting events	.07	.28	25
Total	8.49	17.90	47
All other expenditure	33.89	50.56	67
Total expenditure	42.38	68.46	62
N =	269	364	
Proportion who are women, %	50	50	

HEALTH

In the survey carried out by Age Concern in 1977[2] among 1,640 non-institutionalised people aged 65 or more and living in four English towns respondents were asked if they suffered from any of the 21 ailments contained on a list that ranged from arthritis to incontinence and from high blood pressure to 'breathlessness after even light effort'. Of those aged 65 to 74, 16 percent said they were completely untroubled by any of the 21 impairments but then at the other extreme an equal number said that they suffered from at least four of them with arthritis/rheumatism, backache, giddyness, poor eyesight, and breathlessness being some of the difficulties most commonly mentioned.

Among those aged 75 or more only 10% said they were completely untroubled by any of the listed ailments, but more than twice as many said they suffered from at least four of them; the most commonly mentioned impairments were arthritis/rheumatism, unsteady on feet, poor eyesight, hard of hearing, and forgetfulness. It is hardly surprising that when all respondents were asked: "What would you say makes life really pleasant and satisfying for people of your age"? the second most common response (after 'having good neighbours and friends') was 'Good health'. And in a supplementary question 39% of those nominating 'good health' as the main basis for a satisfying life for elderly people then went on to say that they had good health to a great extent, but 15% said they had it hardly at all or even lacked it completely.

This range of health conditions among the elderly was also found in the *General Household Survey* carried out in 1979.[3] Respondents were asked

> "Do you have any long-standing illness, disability or infirmity? By long-standing I mean anything that has troubled you over a period of time or that is likely to affect you over a period of time.
>
> If YES, does this illness or disability limit your activities in any way?"

'Long-standing illness' was defined as a positive answer to the first part of the question but approximately 40% gave a positive answer to both parts of the question, i.e. said they suffered from a long-standing illness that restricted their activities. The findings, by age and sex, are shown in Table 3.

Given this polarisation of the health conditions of the elderly it is reasonable to expect that it would seem sensible to about half of them if they were urged to pursue a life style that embraced frequent long brisk walks, plenty of gardening, elaborate do-it-yourself jobs round the house and similar strenuous activities; but to another 40% of the elderly advice to do the same would appear to them foolish and irrelevant, and no matter what the state of their health had been in middle age or youth they would be

TABLE 3
INCIDENCE OF LONG-STANDING ILLNESS, BY AGE AND SEX

	Men		Women	
	65 - 74	75 & over	65 - 74	75 & over
	%	%	%	%
No long-standing illness	50	44	48	36
L.S.T., but not limiting	13	11	14	10
Limiting longstanding illness	37	45	38	54
	100	100	100	100

wise in old age to adopt life styles that included large elements of what those devoted to the activity theory of ageing would describe pejoratively as idleness, passivity, self-imposed house-boundness etc. It is worth remembering that in 1979 the 20 hospitals participating in the *Home Accident Surveillance Scheme*[4] recorded 46,200 accidents in which the patient was aged 15 years or more, and of these patients nearly a quarter were aged 65 or more; approximately half these accidents to elderly people were falls and most of the falls suffered by those aged 65 or more occurred in a milieu they were very familiar with - their kitchen or their living room.

USE OF TIME

The most recently published volume of *Social Trends*[5] indicates that very small proportions of the elderly population spend much of their time earning a living. In 1981 the 'economic activity rate' for women over pensionable age (60) was no more than 6.5% and for men over pensionable age (65) the rate was 8.0%; and in both sexes 'economic activity' usually took the form of a part-time job. For all practical purposes we can therefore assume that the average elderly person after allowing a conventional 8 hours each night in bed and four hours each day for getting up, washing and dressing, preparing and eating meals, and washing up, making beds and carrying out similar more or less unavoidable domestic tasks has at his or her disposal 12 hours of leisure time each day seven days of the week, i.e. time they can spend at home watching television, reading, taking a nap, receiving visiting friends and relatives, or out of doors doing the shopping, spending some time at a neighbourhood club, visiting friends and relatives, taking a walk etc. Before looking at some of these activities in detail a broad general picture is provided by a survey carried out in the spring of 1981[6] on behalf of the European Value

Systems Study Group. The questions that bear on the use of time by the elderly were:

Q.1 "Thinking of the way you spend your leisure time, what is more important to you - relaxing as much as possible or doing things, being active?"

The replies show for each age group a marked polarisation of preferences - 3 in 10 opting for a life of relaxation, 5 in 10 preferring activity, and only 2 in 10 choosing what might be considered the more sensible combination of some relaxation and some activity.

TABLE 4

PREFERRED USE OF LEISURE TIME

		Age	
	65 - 74	75 +	All 65 +
	%	%	%
Sitting and relaxing	33	30	32
Doing things	45	52	48
Both equally	22	18	20
	100	100	100
N =	127	82	209

Q.2 "And during your leisure time do you prefer to be alone, to be with your family, to be with friends, or to be in a lively place with many people?" Here the preferences of the young elderly and the old elderly show some divergence. The former, compared with those aged 75 or more, show a marked preference for spending their leisure with family and friends; on the other hand the old elderly are much more desirous of spending their leisure alone.

TABLE 5

PREFERRED COMPANY IN LEISURE TIME

		Age	
	65 - 74	75 +	All 65 +
	%	%	%
Alone	13	28	19
With family	52	33	44
With friends	25	18	22
In a lively place	6	9	7
All equally	4	12	8
	100	100	100

Q.3 "Apart from weddings, funerals and baptisms, about how often do you attend religious services these days"?

This survey, like many others showed that among the total sample of all adults attending any kind of religious service is an extremely rare experience. It is sometimes claimed, however, that this generalisation does not apply to the elderly - in part because religion played a larger part in their childhood upbringing, and in part because as people age they find in religion values and support not available to them in a secular world. The findings of this survey do not support this but do, as with other surveys on religious attendances, show for the elderly, as for all adults, a polarisation of behaviour with one group (admittedly a small one) regular and frequent in its attendances and at the other extreme a group (a larger one) who are almost total strangers to such services.

TABLE 6
ATTENDANCES AT RELIGIOUS SERVICES

	All adults	Adults aged 65 +
	%	%
Once a week or more	14	16
Once a month	9	10
Christmas, Easter etc.	12	11
Once a year	8	8
Less frequently or never	57	55
	100	100

The Age Concern survey[2] of 1977 dealt in some detail with the amount of time spent by elderly people on various activities both at home and out of doors. Some of the findings are summarised in the following tables in the form of averages - and like most averages they hide very considerable differences. For example, on the average day the average person aged 75 or more watched television for 2.9 hours, but 16% of them watched no television, while 18% spent 5 hours or more in front of their sets. Or again, on the average day the average man aged 75 or more spent .60 hours out walking, but this average embraced 61% of them who did not go out for a walk of any duration and 19% who took a walk that filled 2 or more hours.

As far as the time-uses dealt with in Table 7 are concerned the only significant difference between the two age groups relates to the amount of time spent in 'just resting'; the old elderly spent much more time on this than did the young elderly, but even so, this came for both groups a

TABLE 7
TIME SPENT 'YESTERDAY': NO. OF HOURS

	Age		
	65 - 74	75 or more	All 65 +
Watching TV	2.9	2.9	2.9
Listening to radio	1.6	1.4	1.5
Resting	1.6	2.2	1.9
Reading	1.2	1.3	1.2
Going for a walk	.6	.5	.6
Other pastimes*	1.0	.8	.9
	8.9	9.1	9.0

* Football pools, cards etc.

poor second to watching television; sometimes the two activities have a great deal in common.

As part of the survey of elderly life styles respondents were also asked if on the Saturday and Sunday before being interviewed they had gone out of the house at all for any purpose, and if so for what purposes. This probe into venturing out revealed interesting class differences and accordingly Table 8 is presented in terms not only of age but also of class.

TABLE 8
TRIPS OUT LAST WEEKEND

	Age 65 - 74		Age 75 or more	
	Middle class	Working class	M/C	W/C
	%	%	%	%
None	26	36	44	44
1 trip	31	32	22	34
2 trips	33	26	26	18
3 or more	10	6	8	4
	100	100	100	100

In the younger age band the proportion of working class respondents who failed completely to go out was much higher than among middle class respondents. There was no such difference in the older age band, but whereas only 22% of working class men and women went out on at least two occasions the corresponding proportion among middle class respondents was much higher at 34%.

Part of the elderly person's time is taken up by receiving visitors, and to examine this aspect of their leisure they were asked if they had received any visits from friends or relatives during the previous weekend. In both groups over half said they had not. Those who said they had been visited were asked to describe their relationship to their visitors. For both age groups they had been predominantly family relations - offspring and siblings; those over 75 years of age were however more likely than those aged 65 to 74 to be visited by friends.

TABLE 9
"ANY VISITORS LAST WEEKEND"?

		Age 65 - 74	Age 75 +
		%	%
	Yes	42	45
		%	%
Who?	Family	74	65
	Friends	25	34
	Others	1	1
		100	100

It is tempting when going through figures of the kind presented in this paper to attempt in conclusion to draw up a typology of life styles peculiar to elderly people - usually one ranging from complete passivity to manic activity. Probably the two most widely known and useful of these classifications are those constructed by Guillemard[7] and by Havighurst.[8] However I refrain from this since I believe that whatever the losses of the ageing person - of spouse, brothers and sisters, children, job, income, health, etc. - a person's character and values rarely change with advancing years. "The things that have always been important to us remain so, and therefore we must find ways to do things, be the things, have the things that have been important, even in some modified way".[9]

REFERENCES

1. Department of Employment. *Family Expenditure Survey*, 1979.
2. Abrams, M. *Beyond Three Score and Ten*, Age Concern Survey, 1977.
3. Central Statistics Office. *General Household Survey 1979*, HMSO, London, 1982.
4. Home Accident Surveillance Unit Department of Industry. *Home Accident Surveillance Scheme*, 1981.
5. *Social Trends No. 12*. HMSO, 1982.
6. Survey by Social Surveys (Gallup Poll) Ltd., on behalf of the European Value Systems Study Group, 1981.
7. Guillemard, A. *La Retraite - Une Morte Sociale*, Paris, 1972.

8. Havighurst, R. 'Ageing in Western Society' in *The Social Challenge of Ageing*, Hobman, D. (Ed.), London, 1978.
9. Hartford, M. *Today's Research*, University of Southern California Press, 1977.

ADDITIONAL REFERENCE

Abrams, M. 'Changes in the Lifestyles of the Elderly, 1959 to 1982'. *Social Trends 14*, HMSO, London, 1984.

Poverty and Income Maintenance

Siobhan Lloyd

INTRODUCTION

> 'In moving into old age, people tend to separate into two groups, one anticipating a comfortable and even early retirement, the other dreading the prospect and depending almost entirely on the resources made available to it by the state, through its social security system'.[1]

Since the beginning of the twentieth century the number of men over 65 and women over 60 in Britain has increased by more than 300 per cent. These 'elderly' now comprise 16 per cent of the British population. At the same time, taking the state's definition of poverty,* the elderly now comprise 36% of all households with an income at or below the poverty line. Poverty for the elderly, as for other disadvantaged groups, cannot be measured solely in terms of the income made available to individuals and families. The position of an individual in the class structure, for example, is related in turn to command over resources such as savings, interest, employment benefits and access to social services which, together with income, protect social status. For the purpose of this review, and because it provides a more realistic measure of poverty, Townsend's definition will be used as a reference point. He includes in his definition

> 'That section of the population whose resources are so depressed from the mean as to be deprived of enjoying the benefits and participating in the activities which are customary in that society can be said to be in poverty'.[1]

This paper will review the research on poverty as it affects the elderly

* Here the poverty line is defined by the supplementary benefit scale rate appropriate to each family. Those whose household income does not exceed 140 per cent of this minimum are 'on the margins of poverty'.

population, examining studies which question the nature of poverty among the elderly, studies which draw attention to the importance of age, sex and class differences, and studies which examine the various sources of income for the elderly. Research relating to access to resources in housing, employment and social services will be examined, along with the perceptions the elderly themselves have of their own situation. In conclusion, the implications of the research for policy will be explored.

An understanding of the low income and dependency status of the elderly can be gained from a variety of standpoints. It is possible, for example, to explain their economic insecurity by the way in which society's institutional structures promote inequalities in the distribution of income. George[2], for example, finds an explanation in

> 'the dominant economic values of society which dictate that the allocation of goods and services in society must be patterned on people's incomes from work or private resources ... income from the state should not be as great as income from work'.

An advantage of this standpoint is that it concentrates on the causes rather than the consequences of poverty, and, does not therefore hold the risk of researchers searching for the cause of poverty among the supposed inadequacies of the poor themselves. Alternatively there are those writers whose starting point is the shortcomings of the contemporary income maintenance system. Child Poverty Action Group[3], for example, argues that the incomplete implementation of the Beveridge proposals for a national insurance system goes a long way towards accounting for present day poverty among the elderly. An extension of this argument is made by Walker[4] who suggests that because of the terms which are used to justify a fixed and in some ways arbitrary cut off point in an individual's working life, terms such as 'efficiency' and 'productivity' function to confirm the judgement that the elderly can no longer contribute to society's productive activities. Similarly, he argues, the elderly are seen as passive recipients of welfare rather than active participants in a wage orientated society; consequently the idea of chronological age being significant in causing poverty and dependency is rejected in favour of the 'relationship between the social construction of age and the social division of labour' [4] as the cause.

NATURE OF THE RESEARCH

That poverty is widespread among the elderly has long been recognised by both official and independent research from Booth's work[5] at the end of the last century to the most recent official survey in 1966[6]. Hunt[7] however did undertake a major analysis of the living standards of people over sixty-five living in the community for which she used OPCS data. However since Rowntree's pioneering work on poverty in York, researchers have, according to Walker[4] tended to accept the life cycle approach 'as if it were natural law'. It has only comparatively recently been suggested than an explanation for the persistence of poverty in old age can be made by examining the socio-economic status of the elderly within the prevailing social and economic structure. This approach stresses the importance of the three inter-related factors in the explanation of poverty among the elderly: firstly, their social and class position, secondly, the institutional processes which define and create their dependent status and thirdly, the response in the form of social policies to that dependent status. Townsend[1] has added an extra dimension, that 'general propensity to poverty is a function of low levels of resources and restricted access to resources relative to younger people'.

Official research on the subject started with a Royal Commission in 1895[8] which investigated the aged poor and recommended changes in the Poor Law in favour of the elderly. In 1941 the Committee of Inquiry chaired by Sir William Beveridge[9] began to look at the whole system of social security. Its proposals for pensions should be seen against the background for an overall system of insurance covering everyone, whatever their income, and for benefits including pensions to be paid to all those who had contributed to the scheme. In 1953 an official committee chaired by Sir Thomas Phillips[10] was set up to 'review the economic and financial problems involved in providing for old age, having regard to the prospective increase in the numbers of aged and to make recommendations'. The economic problems were identified by the committee as those involving freeing resources from the economy to provide for the elderly, and the financial problems were those arising from the need to transfer to the elderly increased purchasing power so that they could have more command over resources in the economy.

Then in 1965, the Ministry of Pensions and National Insurance,[6] against a growing body of evidence from independent researchers that old people were living on low incomes, carried out a study to establish the extent of the problem and the reasons for elderly people not claiming their entitlements from the National Assistance Board. Over 11,000 elderly people were included in the research, which found that the elderly had 40% lower than average household incomes and that they had very different expenditure patterns to the rest of the population, spending proportionately more on fuel, light, food and housing. The study established that one half of the men in the sample had occupational pensions, compared with one quarter of the single women and one ninth of widows. It also found that more than 700,000 pensioner households could have received more assistance from the National Assistance Board had they applied for it.

There has also been a plethora of reports from independent researchers on the causes and nature of poverty among the elderly, starting with Booth's works in 1892[11] and 1894[5]. Rowntree's[12] early studies of poverty in York, carried out in 1899, 1936 and 1948 concluded that the main causes of poverty were low wages in 1899, unemployment in 1936 and old age in 1948. Rowntree[13] also carried out one of the first large scale social surveys of the elderly between 1944-46. One of the main conclusions of this report was that acute poverty among the elderly had been substantially reduced or even abolished, and that state pensions were adequate. Furthermore the report suggested that there was a certain degree of flexibility within the National Assistance Board since it was able to adjust benefits to meet needs in a reasonably humane way.

Other important national studies began to appear in the late 1950's and early 1960's. Before this time most independent research tended to focus on the medical aspects of ageing; however Walker[4] and others broadened their work to include socio-economic aspects of the subject. Richardson[5] for example in a study of 244 retired men in Aberdeen aged between 65 and 74, was concerned not only to examine the needs and problems of older people, but to answer questions about the importance of social class, geographical factors and socialisation on the elderly.

Cole and Utting[6] published the results of a national study of 4,000 elderly persons in 1962. They looked at problems of loneliness, poverty and ill-health in seven areas. They concluded that the problems were encountered in an acute form by relatively few of their sample and saw the elderly as a largely dependent group with income transferred to them from the economically active population. Among those over retirement age, they wrote, there are three times as many units at the bottom end of income distribution and less than half as many at the top as among the population generally.

Also in 1962/3, Townsend and Wedderburn[7] undertook a national survey of 4,000 elderly people, and found that they had, on average, income levels less than those of younger persons, that few had any assets and that 33% were totally reliant on state benefits. Hunt's[7] study of almost 12,000 elderly people in 90 randomly chosen parliamentary constituencies drew similar conclusions although when asked about particular difficulties they faced, financial issues did not figure prominently in the elderly's own perceptions of their situation. However when asked about ways in which their situation could be improved, some of their suggestions had obvious financial implications. A further importance of Hunt's work was the way it drew attention to differences between the 'young elderly' and very elderly. This was also taken up by Abrams [18] in work undertaken on behalf of Age Concern. He found, for example, that the young elderly have higher material expectations and, that as they age, they are less likely to remain satisfied with their circumstances than the old elderly. Abrams[19] has also used Family Expenditure Survey data and his own research to provide a wealth of information about the living standards of the elderly and their perception of their own situation. Other relevant work by the Age Concern Research Unit includes work on pension incomes[20] and employment in retirement.[21]

One major cross-national study[22] was published in 1968 and produced important material on health and incapacity. Part of the British input to the study[23] identified four major determinants of income in old age; retirement and the contrast between work and no work, economic status during working life, the role of government and, for women, widowhood.

Townsend's[1] major work on the nature and extent of poverty in the United Kingdom provided a wealth of new evidence about the living conditions of the elderly, and challenged conventionally held views about the elderly's dependent status. He suggested that 'there is a dual process of deprivation, stemming fundamentally from class position but also from changing class structure'. The poverty of some old people could be explained, he suggested, with reference to their lifelong low class position. "Others are poor by virtue of society's imposition upon the elderly of an 'underclass' status".

There have also been many smaller local studies which have either looked at the issue of income, poverty, and dependence among the elderly in a specific geographical area[24] or have undertaken action research in respect of specific problems such as non take-up of benefits.[25] Finally there are studies which attempt to determine the causal factors for specific problems such as hypothermia[26] or access to housing.[27]

WHY ARE THE ELDERLY POOR? RESEARCH RELATING TO THE CONSEQUENCES OF RETIREMENT

Why is it that three out of every four households living in poverty contain an elderly person? The Royal Commission on the Distribution of Income and Wealth[7] concluded, 'it is because certain types of individuals are not usually in work that they feature largely in lower levels of income distribution'. This is a key statement when one examines the overriding value which industrialised society places on work.

Retirement, and with it removal from active participation in the labour force, has become a socioeconomic phenomenon of immense importance. Hunt[7] estimated that in 1931 over 50% of men over sixty-five were working; this had declined to 31% by 1951 and by 1971 the figure was 19% (12 % for women).

Loss of income is a major factor determining poverty in old age, and in view of this it is highly questionable whether government policy should encourage retirement through pension rules and limitations on earnings, without providing an adequate pension scheme. The retirement age acts, according to Walker[4], as 'an arbitrary cut off point distinguishing the socially and economically useful from the dependent which is imposed on elderly workers regardless of ability'. Indeed Townsend's recent research [1] suggests that the concept of retirement and its association with particular ages can be explained more by socio-economic considerations than by greater infirmity among the over 60's. He suggests that there is no evidence to suppose that people over 60 or 65 are more infirm than they were in 1908 when means-tested contributory benefits were introduced for people over 70.

It is also important to note that Beveridge's[9] proposals for a national insurance scheme to include the elderly included the principle that pensions were for retirement rather than for old age. He was adamant that 'pensions should be adequate for subsistence without other means, and should be given only to people who, after reaching minimum retirement age have, in fact, retired from work'. In support of this he recommended a retirement rule which would deter people from retirement for as long as possible. This is interesting in the light of current employment policy measures such as the Job Release Scheme which puts pressure on those reaching the later stages of their working life to take early retirement or voluntary redundancy.

The MPNI survey[6] and subsequent research suggested that while many people would prefer to retire early, others, faced with the prospect of a dramatic fall in income in retirement would prefer to stay at work.

Reduced social status on retirement has been identified by Hunt[7] as part of a longer term trend towards rising occupational status with up to twenty years experience of work followed by a slight overall decline. However Walker[4] and Townsend[1] both acknowledge that those who are most vulnerable to loss of employed status at a fixed retirement age are also most likely to suffer redundancy and unemployment at an earlier stage in their working lives. In April 1977 the unemployment rate for men 60 - 64 years was almost double that for all workers, and that figure had doubled since 1971.[28]

WHO ARE THE ELDERLY POOR? RESEARCH RELATING TO AGE, SEX, AND CLASS DIFFERENCES

One in four of all elderly people has an income equal to or below the poverty line, compared to a figure of one in twenty of the non elderly population. The problem is common to both socialist and capitalist societies. Wedderburn, in a British study, established that 23% of elderly couples, 29% of men and half of all aged women in Britain had incomes below the poverty line. Local studies have helped to fill out that national picture, all indicating that poverty among the elderly is more acute in inner city areas and rural areas where traditional industries are in decline.

Coates and Silburn[29] took their poverty line at 20% above supplementary benefit rates, and found in the St. Ann's district of Nottingham that 25.9% of all pensioners had a poverty income. Syson and Young[30], using a similar measure, found that 30.9% of their London sample were living below the poverty line. Butcher and Crosbie[24] in a rural sample of 302 in Cleator Moor, Cumbria showed that one quarter of their respondents had disposable incomes no greater than 120% of the supplementary benefit levels. All of those figures confirm in a dramatic way the vast amount of poverty which exists among the elderly population. Indeed, whatever cut off point is taken, the figures suggest that income poverty is far from a residual problem confronting a minority of the elderly population. On the contrary, low incomes are the lot of a substantial minority.

It is however important to draw attention to internal differences within the elderly population and between the elderly and the rest of the population. Townsend[1] has stressed that much research has focussed on the elderly as independent of the rest of society. Consequently, he argues, the principal causes of poverty have been attributed to individual factors - adjustment problems regarding the ageing process, adjustments to decreasing physical ability and adjustments to retirement.

Recent research however has identified three important areas for consideration, namely the differences between the 'young elderly' and the very aged, differences between the sexes and differences which are attributable to social status.

[i] *The age differences*

The over 75's are the poorest group of all - 53% of them are entitled to supplementary benefit compared with 45% of those in their late sixties. A positive correlation has been established between advancing age and diminishing resources. In addition, the very elderly are less likely to have access to an occupational pension. The very old are hardest hit by inflation, their living accommodation is likely to be most in need of repair and their stock of consumer durables is more likely to be low or in a state of poor repair. Hunt's study[7] showed that while 53% of all elderly households have a washing machine and 75% a fridge, the corresponding figure for the over seventy-fives were 33% and 53%.

Townsend[1] has also indentified the growth of a four generational social structure with a noticeable division among the elderly between the active and the frail and among those who are separated in age by twenty to thirty years. Abrams[18] takes up this point in his 1980 study.

[ii] *Sex differences*

Society makes scant provision for women of pensionable age. Women's position is both a function of age and of lack of, and access to, resources. Abrams[19] in 1977 established that average incomes among the elderly varied from £29.60 for a woman living alone to £56.20 for a married couple. This compared with an average weekly income at the time for an industrial manual worker of £91. Abrams[19] suggested that the poorest household among the elderly is a one person household, the one person being a woman in her mid 70's with no income from employment. The most affluent elderly household contained 2 - 3 persons with one member in employment and the head of the household in her/his mid seventies.

This is confirmed by other research. Cole and Utting[16] suggested that widowed women fared least well of all elderly people, and that women in the lower social classes came out worst of all. A 1966[6] report stated that proportionately more married couples had additional income compared with single or widowed pensioners, and that the proportions without additional income of any kind were consistently and conspicuously higher among single women in all age groups than those found among men, whatever age group.

Reasons for this include the fact that women live longer than men, and are therefore more likely to spend their last years on their own, and that women's wages have been traditionally lower than men's, reducing their potential for saving. In addition the social security system has traditionally operated against women, many of whom have not been economically active in the labour market and have no occupational pension.

Abrams[18] in his study concluded that women living alone were much less likely than other elderly persons to have access to a household washing machine, car, refrigerator, telephone and colour TV set - goods, he suggested which 'could either lighten household chores or increase communication with others'.

[*iii*] *Class differences*

Living standards in old age are also a function of lifelong class position so much so that Townsend[1] concludes 'the elderly poor are an underclass as well as being persons who would be deprived, whatever their age by virtue of their class position'. Higher social status means, among other things, greater eligibility for inheritance and occupational pensions and greater likelihood of home ownership. Walker[4] points out that an implicit reliance by the state on private pensions reinforces class differences among the elderly, since it it less likely that non-manual workers will benefit here. Thus despite redistributive tendencies of state retirement pensions it is most likely that low incomes in retirement will follow low status in working life. The importance of differences in age, sex and class is illustrated when one examines more closely the research which looks at income sources for the elderly.

SOURCES OF INCOME FOR THE ELDERLY: RESEARCH RELATING TO STATE PENSIONS, OCCUPATIONAL PENSIONS AND ASSETS

Regardless of the age when it occurs, a sudden drop in income is the major difficulty involved in moving from work to retirement. This transition involves not only having to live at a lower standard than that previously enjoyed, but also perhaps means joining the ranks of one of the poorest sections of society. Wedderburn[23] suggests that the change in income for persons moving from employment to retirement might properly be described as 'severance rather than a process of income maintenance'.

Townsend[1] has estimated that income on retirement can fall by as much as 50% for a married couple and by 70% for a single person. The wry comment made by one female pensioner, that 'retirement means twice as much husband or half as much income'[31] is true for the greater proportion of the elderly population. Abrams[19] has identified five household types among the elderly (see table 1 below) and, whilst acknowledging the heterogeneity of circumstances in each, he concludes that 'all types of elderly household have substantially lower average incomes than the average for households where the head is not a retired person'.

[*i*] *State benefits*

The first distinctive characteristic of all elderly households is their dependence on state benefits. Overall this constitutes 45% of total income and for some it reaches 60%. Table 1 taken from Abram's research, shows income derived from different sources for the main household types.

The most widely received government benefit in terms of the numbers who receive it and its total amount is retirement pension, yet this has never exceeded the level of supplementary benefit. Therefore any pensioner who is reliant solely on the government pension automatically has an income below that of the government's own defined subsistence level. Between 1948 and 1975 the retirement pension only improved from 30.5 to 31.5% of average male manual earnings, leaving the relative position virtually unchanged. Many people are eligible for supplementary benefit to augment their retirement pension. In Cleator Moor 50% of pensioner households were entitled but nearly one third of those eligible failed to apply.[24] The most important evidence of non-take up of benefits come from Cole and Utting[16] and prompted the government to

TABLE 1

SOURCES OF HOUSEHOLD INCOMES[1] OF THE ELDERLY AND NON-RETIRED

Type of household	Average total weekly household income	Persons in household	Income per head	Sources of income: Wages and salaries	Self employment	Investments	Annuities, private pensions	Social security benefit	Other[2]
	£		£	%	%	%	%	%	%
1 male, 65 or over	25.48	1.0	25.48	10	1	16	18	49	6 = 100%
1 female, 60 or over	22.77	1.0	22.77	9	*	13	10	60	8
1 male and 1 female, head 65 or over	42.70	2.0	21.35	19	3	12	15	46	5
Head of household retired	34.63	1.6	21.50	19	1	12	13	49	6
Head of household 65 or over	37.86	1.7	22.68	24	2	11	12	45	6
1 adult 65 or over	22.27	1.0	22.27	6	1	13	11	62	7
All households where head[3] not retired	84.31	3.2	26.51	81	6	3	1	5	4

1 All income figures in the FES are 'gross', ie, before deduction of income tax, national insurance etc.
2 Other = includes subletting and imputed income from owner/rent-free occupancy.
3 The *not* retired includes those where head of household is unemployed.
* = less than 0.5%.

carry out its own survey of 11,000 elderly[6]. This showed that 750,000 were failing to claim their benefit and led to a replacement of national assistance by a system of supplementary pensions. Townsend[1] argues however that non-take up is not so much due to ignorance about rights, or a reluctance to exercise them, as in administrative difficulties of access to the system.

This issue of non-take up was explored by an action research project in Wandsworth in 1975/6[25]. The project made an in-depth comprehensive survey of the elderly to investigate the knowledge and perception of welfare benefits and the extent of take up. The starting point for the project was a belief that 'the need for money overshadows the more complex social, psychological and physical problems of old age'. The research showed that non-take up is the result of a combination of inter-related factors, including ignorance - of the existence of benefit and about procedure for claiming - the complexity of the forms and the stigma attached to claiming. This is verified by Abrams[18] who also included the dimension of pride felt by many elderly people when it comes to living within their received income.

That elderly people rely overwhelmingly on the state has been confirmed. However if we examine the relative importance of other sources of income and access to resources in retirement at opposite ends of the spectrum of distribution, we can see how it compares with access to resources earlier in the life cycle. Hunt[17] has looked first at those couples with a net income of less than £1,500 per annum. Ninety-eight per cent received a national insurance pension, 35% received some annuity income from shares, property and savings, 46% received an occupational pension, 22% received supplementary benefit and 8% received a wage or salary. For those couples with an income of more than £3,000, 75% received a retirement pension, 92% an annuity income, 68% an occupational pension and none were in receipt of supplementary benefit.

[*ii*] *Occupational pensions*

A secondary source of income is occupational pension, access to which depends on a complex interaction of age, sex and former occupational status. In 1979 over half the workforce was covered by the scheme but not all those currently in retirement qualify. In addition, many elderly women, because of poor paid employment record are not included and in 1978 for those who were in receipt of an occupational pension the average amount received was less than £10 per week.[17] The Cleator Moor study [24] found that half of all retired men but few women were in receipt of occupational pensions, doubtless due to the nature of the former industrial base of the area. Pensions may be indexed linked but they do not improve standards of living because a greater proportion of this income goes on living expenses such as heating and clothing.[32] A further important factor is that although the level of occupational pensions may be low, it is often enough to put its recipients just above the level for claiming supplementary benefit, so excluding them from receiving the other benefits this in turn confers.

The impact of retirement on economic activity rates has already been noted. Townsend[1] has identified additional factors contributing to these rates, namely scientific and technological advances, changes in the industrial structure, high levels of unemployment and the pursuit of economic growth.

[*iii*] *Employment*

Abrams[18] noted that only 4% of men over 65 named employment as their main source of income, while Hunt[17] has estimated that 5.7% of all non-married women and 10% of non-married men over retirement age were in employment. Showler[21] has stressed the importance of the availability of employment to the older person as a determinant of general welfare while a recent *Employment Gazette* report[33] on compulsory retirement concluded that 'if given the chance to stay on, nearly two-thirds would do so'.

The importance of part-time work to the elderly has been stressed by Walker[4] who points out that, while few pre-retirement working males work part-time (up to 30 hours per week) two-thirds of those working post retirement do so. Similarly among women, where 30% of those working pre-retirement are in part-time work, the figure jumps to 80% working part-time post retirement. Families as a main source of income have not been significant. Abrams[19] notes that no men and few women mentioned money from their children as the main source of income, but 14% of men over 75 and 8% of women of the same age get something from their children.

[*iv*] *Assets*

Moore and Butcher[34] have estimated that at the end of 1975 there were

842,000 elderly persons with no capital assets and 352,000 with savings totalling less than £2,000. Townsend[1] paints a bleaker picture. In his sample, 25% had no assets or less than £25 while 20% had assets amounting to less than £22. From this he draws two conclusions: that even when potential assets are counted, a substantial number of the elderly remain on the margins of poverty; however for a small proportion of the elderly, their situation may be transformed from that of having a low or modest income to becoming relatively rich.

In an Age Concern study[27] just over half the sample had capital of less than £325, "Just enough to bury me". Indeed more than one person was so concerned that they went without clothes and blankets rather than use savings they had set aside for their funerals. These findings have been confirmed by Hunt[7] who found that one fifth of elderly couples and a quarter of non-married elderly had less than £300 in assets. Twenty-one percent had an annual income of less than £1,500 and assets of less than £300, while only 6% of all elderly households had an annual income of more than £3,000 and assets of more than £2,500.

[*v*] *Access to other resources*

Although Townsend[1] found that more elderly than non elderly own their own homes, there were also more in privately rented accommodation, indicating more polarisation in housing conditions among the elderly. Added to this, the fact that a higher proportion of elderly people live in pre-1919 housing has suggested a positive correlation with ill-health since 'chronic sickness is more common among people living without heating, a fixed bath and without a lavatory' [1]. In the Cleator Moor study[24] 75% of the sample were found to be without sole use of a w.c., bath or hot running water.

Relative to income the elderly receive more than younger members of society in the value of social services in kind. However this does not reflect additional need since more elderly people are sick and disabled. The fact that they may get more from the National Health Service does not mean that they have a higher standard of living but that they are freed from extra costs.

In Birmingham in 1969, 40% of those studied lived in temperatures of under 60%F[35]. Wicks[26] in a 1972 study of 1,000 elderly concluded that there are 6,000 deaths due to hypothermia a year and that a further 70,000 persons are at risk. He also suggested that elderly married couples in the low income band are four times more likely not to heat their bedrooms. One of the aims of his study was to explore the relationship between poverty and low temperatures, but he found the latter was not in turn associated with income. Nor did his study indicate whether recipients of supplementary benefit are living in colder homes than other pensioners.

[vi] *The effect of low income on expenditure*

Living at or around supplementary benefit levels imposes severe financial restrictions on the lifestyle of the elderly. As income diminishes, more is spent on the essentials of life. Abrams[19] demonstrates that where the head of household is retired and pensionable, then 57% of income goes on food, fuel and housing. For the poorer elderly 72% of income is absorbed in this way.

TABLE 2
EXPENDITURE ON COMMODITY OR SERVICES AS A PERCENTAGE OF TOTAL HOUSEHOLD EXPENDITURE 1975

	Housing	Fuel	Food	Total household expenditure on Food & Fuel	Other expenditure
One Adult					
Men 65 +	20.7	9.2	26.3	56.9	43.1
Women 60 +	23.7	10.2	26.4	60.3	39.1
Man & Woman					
Head of household 65 +	16.8	8.3	27.7	53.8	47.2
All households	13.1	5.5	24.8	43.4	56.6

Source: *Family Expenditure Survey 1975* Table 33, HMSO 1976.

HOW DO THE ELDERLY PERCEIVE THEIR SITUATIONS?

Not surprisingly there is a marked difference in perception between those living on an adequate income and those living at or below supplementary benefit level as there is between the young elderly and very elderly population. Among the over 65s Abrams[36] found that two-thirds of his sample thought they had enough money to get along while 1 in 4 said they couldn't make ends meet. Fifty-three per cent felt secure in relation to their future financial position, while 33% did not express this sense of security.

Abrams asks what it means when two-thirds of the respondents say they have enough to get along. When asked if they felt that present sources of income gave security for the future, 60% of over 75s said yes and 50% of 65 - 74 year olds said no.

In a later study Abrams[18] asked the elderly how much extra would be needed in order to live without money worries and in reasonable comfort. For 57% the answer was 'nothing'. However for those who did acknowledge the need for more, the things they identified needing most were heating, (31%) food (28%) and clothing (12%). When asked how they would describe their present financial position 66% said they had enough to live on, 7% couldn't make ends meet and 27% were 'comfortable'. There was also a high level of material satisfaction amongst those living alone, but when account was taken of their material position it was noted that those living alone tended to have more modest aspirations and expectations and therefore higher levels of satisfaction may have been more easily attained. He also found an interesting comparison between the 64 - 74 age group and those over 75, with the younger age group expressing more dissatisfaction with future prospects. Shelgrove's findings[37] augment these results. From a sample in Luton he recorded the terms used to describe feelings post retirement. Forty-five per cent of respondents said they were 'sad', 'worried', 'anxious', 'lost', or 'bored', 10% were 'resigned' and 12% were 'fed up'. He also found that after retirement only 3.6% were able to say that their income was sufficient, and when asked what sorts of things they had to give up, 66% cited clothes, holidays and home fittings, 33% entertainment and 10% gifts and newspapers. As one of them put it, 'it was a means test every day. We had to cut and cut and cut'.

To conclude, Wicks[26] states quite bluntly that, from the evidence in his research

> 'people in this group are amongst the poorest in Britain. Events that most people take in their stride - shoe repairs, the need to buy a new saucepan ... can seriously affect life at the margin'.

POLICY AND PRACTICE IMPLICATIONS OF THE RESEARCH

The wider policy implications for the research are clear. As far as income support is concerned, there are good grounds for index linking all sources of income for the elderly so that their modest standards of living can be maintained if not improved. Lister[38] has argued for a basic pension level set and index linked at no less than 60% of average male industrial earnings. Walker[4] has argued that to eradicate poverty among the elderly is not simply a matter of providing pensions but rather a question of changing the relationship between age and the labour market, between dependent and independent status and thereby changing the relationship between work and rewards. He has also argued forcibly that positive social policy should not continue to be age-orientated but should be directed towards the institutionalised structures of society, especially in the labour market. Abrams[19] advocates more research into what social conditions are most likely to produce 'pseudo family relationships' for those elderly whose children have moved away. He also quotes one outstanding deprivation expressed by many elderly people - their inability to take holidays, and advocates the development of Elderhostels and Villages de Vacances modelled on European examples.

As is evident from the review of research studies considered, it is important that policies directed at the elderly are not considered in isolation from the prevailing socio-economic climate. The signs are, if the Government White Paper *Growing Older*[39] is to provide an indication of possible future trends in policy, that the 'New Right' will afford little comfort for the elderly poor. This is particularly so in the light of the statement in the White Paper that it is only by controlling inflation that better standards of living for the elderly can be ensured.

REFERENCES

1. Townsend, P. *Poverty in the United Kingdom*. Penguin, London, 1979.
2. George, V. *Social Security and Society*. Routledge and Kegan Paul, London, 1973.
3. Field, F. *Poverty, the facts*. Child Poverty Action Group Poverty Pamphlet No. 21, 1975.
4. Walker, A. 'Poverty and the social creation of dependency in old age'. *Journal of Social Policy*, 9(1), 1980.
5. Booth, A. *The aged poor: Condition*. Macmillan, London, 1894
6. Ministry of Pensions and National Insurance. *Financial and other circumstances of retired pensioners*. MPNI, HMSO, 1966.
7. Hunt, A. *The elderly at home: a study of people aged 65 and over living in the community in England and Wales*. OPCS, HMSO, 1978.
8. *Royal Commission on the Aged Poor*. HMSO, 1895.
9. Beveridge, W. *Social Insurance and Allied Services*. HMSO, London, 1942.
10. Chancellor of the Exchequer. *Report of the committee on the economic and financial problems of the provision for old age*. CMND 9333, HMSO, 1954.
11. Booth, C. *A picture and the endowment of old age: an argument*. Macmillan, London, 1892.

12. Rowntree, S. & Havers, G.R. *Poverty and the Welfare State: A Third Social Survey of York dealing only with economic questions.* Longmans, London, 1951.
13. Rowntree, S. *Old People. Report of a survey committee on the problems of ageing and the care of old people.* The Nuffield Foundation, Oxford University Press, 1947.
14. Walker, K. *Commentary on age.* Jonathan Cape, London, 1952.
15. Richardson, I.M. *Age and need: A study of older people in North East Scotland.* Livingstone, Edinburgh, 1964.
16. Cole, D. & Utting, J. *The economic circumstances of old people.* Codicote Press, 1962.
17. Townsend, P. & Wedderburn, D. *The aged in the Welfare State.* Bell and Sons, London, 1965.
18. Abrams, M. *Beyond three score and ten. Second report on a survey of the elderly.* Age Concern, London, 1980.
19. Abrams, M. *Profiles of the elderly: their standards of living.* Age Concern, London, 1979.
20. Hewitt, P. *Age Concern on pensions and income.* Age Concern, London, 1970.
21. Showler, B. *Employment in Retirement.* Age Concern, London, 1974.
22. Shanas, E, et al. *Old people in three industrialised societies.* Routledge & Kegan Paul, London, 1968.
23. Wedderburn, D. *The financial resources of older people* in Shanas E., et al, 1968.
24. Butcher, H. & Crosbie, D. *Pensioned off: a study of the needs of the elderly in Cleator Moor.* Papers in Community Studies, No. 15., Department of Social Administration, York University, 1977.
25. Pensioners Rights Project Association. *Old proud and poor. Action research project on elderly people and welfare benefits in Wandsworth.* Wandsworth Task Force, 1978.
26. Wicks, M. *Old and Cold.* Heinemann, London, 1978.
27. Age Concern. *Housing and finance: a survey of elderly people's housing circumstances and related benefits.* Age Concern, London, 1974.
28. Beveridge, Sir W. *Social Insurance and Allied Social Services.* HMSO, 1942.
29. Layard, R., Piachaud, D., & Stewart, M. *The causes of poverty.* Background paper No. 5. Royal Commission on the Distribution of income and wealth. HMSO, 1978.
30. Coates, K. & Silburn, R. *Poverty, the forgotten Englishman.* Penguin, London, 1970.
31. Syson, L. & Young, M. 'Poverty in Bethnal Green' in Young, M. (Ed) *Poverty Report,* Temple Smith, 1974.
32. Search Project. *Against Ageism.* Search Project, Newcastle, 1981.
33. Lewis, P. 'Pensions, inflation and savings' in Lewis, P. et al. *Inflation and low incomes.* Fabian Research, Series 322, 1975.
34. Commentary in Emloyment Gazette, January, 1981.
35. Butcher, H. & Moore. *The Xmas Bonus.* Poverty Pamphlet, 28, Child Poverty Action Group, 1974.
36. Harling, J. & Gullick, S. *A study of living conditions among the aged in Birmingham.* Wallace Friendship Fund, 1969.
37. Abrams, M. *Beyond three score and ten. A first report on a survey of the elderly.* Age Conern, London, 1978.
38. Shelgrove, D.R. *Elderly employed: a report on elderly people who are in employment.* White Crescent Press, 1965.
39. Lister, R. *Social Security, the case for reform.* Child poverty Action Group Pamphlet 22, 1975.
40. Department of Health and Social Security. *Growing Older.* CMND 8713, HMSO, 1981.

ADDITIONAL REFERENCES

Altmann, R.M. 'Incomes of the early retired'. *Journal of Social Policy*, 11,3, 1982.
(A study of incomes of men retiring before the age of 65.)

Bradshaw, J. & Harris, T. *Energy and Social Policy*. Routledge & Kegan Paul, London, 1983,
(Examines aspects of energy policy, the extent of fuel poverty and the resultant problem of hypothermia.)

Creedy, J. *State Pensions in Britain*. Cambridge University Press, Cambridge, 1982.
(Examines state pensions in Britain with particular reference to the new state pension scheme introduced in 1978.)

Estes, C.L. & Newcomer, R.J. *Fiscal Austerity and Ageing and Shifting Government Responsibility for the Elderly*. Sage, London & Beverly Hills, 1983.
(A look at past and present social policy towards the elderly in the U.S. and the fiscal conditions of state and local government.)

Guillemard, A. (ed.) *Old Age and the Welfare State*. Sage Studies in International Sociology (2B).
(A comparative study of the relationship between policy towards the ageing and class structure, economics and the state apparatus of the U.S., Canada, U.K., Italy, W. Germany and France.)

Irving, D. 'How statistics can plot areas of need'. *Health and Social Services Journal*. No. 4869, 20:10:83.
(A look at some of the indicators which can be used to measure deprivation among elderly people.)

James, C. *Occupational Pensions: the Failure of Private Welfare*. Fabian Society, 1984.
(Documents the evidence for the failure of occupational pensions to meet need in old age.)

Judge, K. 'Private insurance or social security?' *Yearbook of Social Policy*, 1983. Jones, K. & Stevenson, J. (eds.), Routledge & Kegan Paul, 1984.
(Examines the choices facing those in employment in relation to private pension schemes.)

Kerr, S. *Making Ends Meet: an Investigation into the Non Claiming of Supplementary Pensions*. Bedford Square Press, London, 1983.

Parker, H. *Action on Welfare: the Reform of Personal Income Taxation and Social Security*. Social Affairs Unit, 1984.
(Examines the reform of social security and the personal taxation system.)

Phillipson, C. *Capitalism and the Social Construction of Old Age*. Macmillan, London, 1982.

Rose, E. A. — *Housing Needs and the Elderly*. Gower, Aldershot, 1982.
(Research carried out to identify and critically assess the extent of unmet needs for housing and ancillary factors for older people in Birmingham.)

Smith, W. — *Inflation and Elderly People*. Age Concern, Mitcham, 1982.

Stace, S. & Lees, A. — *Hope and Despair: Elderly People in London's Docklands*. Age Concern, London, 1983.
(A research report on the socio-economic conditions of elderly people in the Docklands of London. Report presented to London Dockland Corporation.)

Taylor, G. — 'Cold comfort'. *Nursing Times*, 78,5, 1982.
(Statistics on the incidence of hypothermia.)

Taylor, R. & Ford, G. — 'Inequalities in old age: an examination of age, sex and class differences in a sample of community elderly'. *Ageing and Society*, 3,2, July 1983.
(The distribution of personal resources between age cohorts, sex groups and social classes in a random sample of community elderly.)

Walker, A. — 'Dependency and old age'. *Social Policy and Administration*, 16,2, 1982.

Working Party Report — *Fuel Hardship: towards a Social Policy*. Report compiled by a working party of AMS, ACC, ADC, COSLA, LBA. London, 1982.
(Report examining problems faced by low income households in paying for fuel.)

Sheltered Housing

Hans Wirz

THE DEMOGRAPHIC CONTEXT

Population projections show that the elderly constitute a large and increasing proportion of the population.

In 1979 almost 14% of the Scottish population were over the age of 65, a total of some 718,000 people, and this figure has grown to 726,100.[1] Furthermore, significant changes within the age structure of the elderly are taking place. As the SHHD/SED *Care of the Elderly Report*[2] puts it, 'the elderly population is itself aging'. Up to 1991 the number of people aged 65 - 74 is expected to decline while those over 75 and over 85 is expected to increase. This projected increase in the number of people over 75 has implications for the planners of health and social services; as Bosanquet says, 'it is usually held that a person over 75 uses eight times more health and social services than the normal equivalent adult' [3].

Another important factor which is likely to influence the demand on services is the large number of elderly who live alone. The 1971 census showed that 25% of persons of pensionable age lived alone, compared to 16% in 1961. The number of single person households is expected to increase by 35% from 1978 to 1991,[4] and the number of single elderly households is expected to increase by 27% over the same period.

If one adds to the above figures the fact that as a group the elderly often live in the worst housing, as was for instance shown in Gruer's study[5], the size of the problem begins to emerge.

THE SIZE OF 'THE PROBLEM'

According to a report published by the Scottish Federation of Housing

Associations,[6] there are some 40 applicants for each available sheltered flat. This figure is almost certainly an underestimate and is likely to increase as the benefits of sheltered housing become more widely known. Table I published in the above report[7] shows the shortfall by Region.

TABLE I
SHELTERED HOUSING NEEDED TO MEET MINIMUM STANDARD[8]
[50 UNITS/1000 ELDERLY]

Region	% of minimum needs provided	No. of extra houses required
Borders	44%	510
Central	33%	1,160
Dumfries	13%	950
Fife	10%	1,880
Grampian	35%	2,190
Highland	28%	930
Lothian	26%	3,970
Strathclyde	19%	13,350
Tayside	52%	1,500
Islands	50%	300
Scotland	26%	26,720

A more detailed analysis of these figures shows that in only one of the 56 Housing Districts in Scotland, i.e. the Shetland Islands, is there adequate provision of sheltered housing, using SDD's own criteria of 50 units per 1000 elderly.[9]

Comparisons with England and Wales are also unfavourable. Butler[10] reckoned that approximately 5% of the elderly were in sheltered housing in England and Wales, whereas a recent Scottish study[11] estimates that only 1.6% of the population over pensionable age in Scotland is at present in sheltered housing.

The need is therefore great and urgent, since 'unlike some other priority groups, the elderly do not have time on their side. All too often their plight goes unnoticed and is unheard in the determining of base local and national priorities'.[12]

THE DEVELOPMENT OF SHELTERED HOUSING IN SCOTLAND

Sheltered housing has been developed as part of a strategy to meet the housing needs of the elderly. It is a relatively new form of provision, which has become available more slowly in Scotland than in England. Sumner and Smith[13] felt that this was a product of the different legislative framework, which meant that until 1964 welfare authorities in Scotland were not empowered to make financial contributions to housing authorities for sheltered housing. In 1970 the *Scottish Housing Handbook,* Bulletin 3,[14] laid down design standards which distinguished between Special Housing for the more active elderly and Sheltered Housing for the frailer elderly.

In Type 1, or Special Housing, facilities such as common room and warden service could be provided but were not obligatory. Sheltered Housing, or Type 2, had to have a resident warden and facilities such as a common room, laundry and guest rooms.

However, over a period of time, problems arose in maintaining the distinction between the two types of scheme. Many active elderly living in Type 1 schemes became frail and needed extra support which was not available . A further difficulty was caused by the need to supply certain mandatory facilities in sheltered housing which made schemes costly, regardless of the extent to which they were needed or would be used by the tenants.

In 1975 the Scottish Office issued Circular No. 120/1975[15] which introduced a more flexible approach to the provision of housing for the elderly. The distinction between the above two types of housing was abolished and sheltered housing was now defined as specially designed housing for the elderly which met certain basic design standards. Those features of sheltered housing, such as heated corridors, common rooms and laundries which were once mandatory became optional. This permitted local authorities and housing associations to choose the mix of facilities which they could provide in individual developments once certain mandatory features were included. The above circular stated that sheltered housing is one of three types of housing for the elderly, the other two being labelled as mainstream and amenity housing. This recognises that many dwellings in the general housing stock, particularly small ones, are suitable for the elderly i.e. mainstream housing. However, some elderly require accommodation designed specifically to meet their needs and when this incorporates whole house heating, grab rails and special bathroom fittings, it is known as amenity housing. Add a warden, an alarm system and some other optional facilities, and it becomes sheltered housing.

The years since the publication of the circular have seen a rapid expansion in the provision of sheltered housing in Scotland, and housing associations in particular have been active in this field. Clark[16], in a report published by the Scottish Federation of Housing Associations, states that sheltered housing has become a focus of housing association activity and accounts for over 50% of housing associations new building development.

RESEARCH IN THE FIELD OF SHELTERED HOUSING

The growing interest in sheltered housing is reflected by the number of recent research projects, particularly in England and Wales, although some of these studies were restricted to specific housing associations, while others were limited to sheltered housing within small local areas. The main focus of some of the studies was to obtain more information about the tenants of the schemes, but others, such as Boldy's[17] also examined the role of the warden in sheltered housing. A comprehensive study of sheltered housing in England and Wales has recently been undertaken by the University of Leeds[18], which looked at provisions in twelve local authority housing areas. However, the studies in England and Wales are of limited relevance to Scotland, although it is of interest in many instances to try and make comparisons.

A similar study[11], covering a sample of 33 schemes within 5 districts of Scotland, including a rural district in the north of Scotland, one in the Borders, a New Town and 2 districts from the Central Belt, has recently been completed and in the remainder of this article a selection of the findings of this study will be presented. A sample of tenants and households were interviewed, together with all the wardens of the 33 schemes. Furthermore, GPs, health board and social work staff were asked their views of sheltered housing by way of a self-completion questionnaire.

THE SCOTTISH STUDY[11] *- A SELECTION OF FINDINGS*

A profile of the residents

In order to ascertain if the benefits of sheltered housing are reaching those households for which it is intended, a variety of information was obtained on the social characteristics of the residents in the schemes in the study.

Household composition and age

The overwhelming majority of households were single people - mainly single women. The household composition of respondents is set out below in Table II.

TABLE II

Household type	Percentage
Single men	11
Single women	66
Married couples	22
Pairs of sisters/ Brother and sister	1
	100%
	(N = 226)

Women were over-represented when compared to the elderly in general and although the age of sheltered housing tenants in the sample varied from 53 to 93 the average age was 75 years old and the proportion aged over 75 was substantially higher than the general population of pensionable age.

Incomes

Most households in the sample were dependent on state benefits - 90% received the state retirement pension and 52% were also in receipt of the state supplementary pension; only 9% received neither the supplementary pension nor rent and rate rebates. Consequently, incomes were generally low - very few had a weekly household income of over £55 and 77% of households had an income of less than £45 per week from all sources (1979). In general, tenants in housing association projects had somewhat higher incomes than those in local authority schemes.

Previous housing

Forty-one per cent of respondents had lived previously in the publicly rented sector, 30% in privately rented or tied housing and 18% in owner-occupied housing. This suggests that owner-occupiers were under-represented in comparison with elderly households in general, but there was a slightly higher percentage of ex-owner-occupiers in housing association schemes than local authority and New Town Development Corporation schemes. A small proportion of respondents had previously lived in houses lacking basic amenities (16% in a house lacking a bathroom, 5% lacking an inside WC). Just over half of the households in the sample had previously lived in housing with 2 or more bedrooms in which they had either lived alone or with their spouse alone. This suggests that a move to sheltered housing can often release possible under-occupied accommodation for those in need of more space. Finally, 66% of respondents had previously lived in dwellings with stairs and almost half (47%) had had difficulty in climbing stairs. Most tenants (87%) had no problems in moving from their previous home; the two types of problems that were reported were the cost of the move and disposal of excess furniture.

Self-reported health problems

Respondents were asked about their physical health and mobility. The percentage of respondents/spouses and tenants reporting particular health problems are set out in Table III.

TABLE III

Health problem	Percentage
Arthritis/rheumatism	48
Poor eyesight	40
Bad hearing	36
Giddiness	31
Heart trouble	27
High blood pressure	20
Headaches	12
	(N = 269)

The under 70s were more likely than the 70 - 84 year olds to assess their health as 'poor' (45% compared with 22%). There are a number of possible interpretations of this result. The older age group may have different standards (having become more accustomed to ill health) or allocation policy may have changed over time (with more opportunity at the outset to establish between frail and fitter tenants). Another possible interpretation is that the younger tenants were admitted because of their relatively poor health, but once in sheltered housing with no more stairs to climb, whole house heating, regular attention and care, their condition stabilised or improved.

Performance of basic tasks

Well over 90% of respondents were able to perform without difficulty basic tasks such as washing and feeding themselves and going to the lavatory. Smaller percentages were able to bath without difficulty (72%), to use public transport without difficulty (64%) and to get up and down stairs (41%). However, there was a considerable degree of similarity between the findings of this survey on ability to perform tasks and information obtained from a national cross sample of the elderly carried out by OPCS[19]. The marked difference was in the percentage of respondents who had difficulty in climbing stairs (59%) - compared with only 33% of the national sample.

Movement out of sheltered housing

It is perhaps often assumed that sheltered housing is an 'intermediate' form of accommodation, somewhere between the independence of an ordinary tenancy or owner-occupation and the care provided in an institution such as an old people's home or geriatric ward, and that tenants in sheltered housing will therefore move on to other accommodation as they become frailer and require more support.

The Scottish study suggests that this assumption is not supported by the data collected, shown in Table IV. This table refers to the total number of vacancies which have occurred in the sample of the Scottish study over the period during which these schemes had been in operation and the reasons for them. These periods varied from ten years to eighteen months.

It appears therefore that for two-thirds of all tenants, sheltered housing is a final form of accommodation. Planners and providers of care for the elderly cannot count on there being a steady turnover, particularly in the early years after a scheme has first opened. It is also worth pointing out that tenants in sheltered housing enjoy the same security of tenure as any other tenants, and should therefore not be regarded like residents of, say,

TABLE IV

Reason for vacancy	Percentage
Death	67
Residential home	11
Hospital	8
Live with relatives	6
Mainstream housing	6
Other	2
	100%
	(N = 217)

an old people's home, who in certain circumstances could be asked to move to accommodation where more intensive care is available. Instead, it seems that the majority, once in sheltered housing, do not move again, but attract an increasing proportion of the various support services.

Overall satisfaction with sheltered housing

Over 90% of the respondents said that they were satisfied with their accommodation. In terms of tenant satisfaction, it is clear that sheltered housing is an overwhelming success. Only 16% of all respondents stated that they would have preferred to remain in their previous house, mainly because of long established ties with the area. Important though the presence of a warden and the existence of an alarm system are to the concept of sheltered housing, it also appeared that the factors which most accounted for the high level of satisfaction related to the tenants' new housing conditions as compared to those previously 'enjoyed' (or, in many cases, more appropriately 'suffered'). This comment is made, not in order to detract from the importance of the warden service or alarm system, since the knowledge that they are there in case of emergency provides immeasurable peace of mind to many, but it does raise the question as to how many relatively fit elderly could have their lot considerably improved by the provision of, say, more amenity housing.

Alarm systems

The alarm system allows the tenant to summon help in case of difficulty. Two-way speech systems were used in 25 of the 33 schemes and the remaining 8 used bell alarms. Wardens generally felt that the two-way or intercom systems tended to be more reliable or easier to operate than the bell systems.

Some 76% of households reported that they had not used the alarm in an emergency within the last year and 12% had only done so once. Given the importance of alarms in the concept of sheltered housing, this relatively low usage may seem surprising. However, as mentioned above, their value should not be judged solely on the amount of usage, rather it lies in the reassurance and peace of mind their availability provided.

The wardens - background and qualifications

Since the issue of the SDD Circular No. 120/1975[21] the critical features of a sheltered housing development have been defined to be a mandatory warden and alarm system.

The typical sheltered housing warden in the sample was middle aged, married and female. The average age was 51 and their ages ranged from 35 to 68. Over 90% were female. The wardens had spent an average of 3.2 years doing the job and time in post ranged from 3 months to 9 years. All but 3 wardens lived in the scheme. Almost half had neither formal academic qualifications nor any professional qualifications, a third of the wardens had a nursing qualification and one warden had a residential social work qualification. Despite the lack of formal qualifications, the wardens had a variety of previous experience of working with elderly people including looking after aged relatives or friends, voluntary work with the elderly, nursing and work in a residential home.

There are a number of indications from the Scottish study that the wardens are performing a very valuable task. Firstly, it is clear that they play a critical role in dealing with emergencies and, although these may not occur frequently, without a warden the only source of help would be other tenants. Secondly, it is clear that wardens provide a source of advice and assistance in getting services and help from outside. Although some tenants might manage this without either advice or assistance, this is unlikely to be generally true. A good warden who is both closely in touch with the day-to-day position of the elderly residents and also well informed about how to seek out and obtain support services if they are required, may well be able to prevent many crises from occurring. It is clear that wardens are often involved in providing direct care in certain situations.

The position of warden in a sheltered housing scheme is a relatively new form of occupation and there is inevitably some lack of clarity about the job. However, there is now a degree of experience to build on and the research indicates a need for a greater awareness of the warden's role. For many wardens, particularly new wardens, a clear specification of duties would be welcomed. It is also important to ensure that both tenants and other professional staff who come into contact with sheltered housing schemes - GPs, social workers, home help etc. - have a clear understanding of the role of the warden.

The newness of the warden role is also reflected in the diversity of their working conditions, both in terms of hours worked, holidays etc. and also in relation to training and support for wardens in their work. There are many inevitable pressures for a warden, both living and working in a sheltered housing scheme, which can lead to ever increasing demands made on their time. Some attempt at a standardisation of working conditions and the development of both pre-service and in-service training might help both to improve job satisfaction and the quality of the service.

Sheltered housing in the community

One of the major policy goals behind the encouragement of sheltered housing is the retention of elderly persons in the 'community' who might otherwise require institutional care. It was therefore thought to be important to examine the links between sheltered housing tenants and the wider community and, in particular, the level and types of domiciliary services required by residents.

Social contacts

It is generally agreed that the siting and allocation of sheltered housing should, where possible, prevent people from being taken out of their community unless at their own request. Over 87% of households moved within the local authority district in which they had previously lived, although, due to the size of some of the districts covered, this may still create problems as even relatively short distances can be a handicap for the elderly. Maintaining contact with family and relatives is also important. Some 88% of respondents were visited by relatives and over three-fifths of those were visited at least once a week. Most frequent visitors were the sons and daughters (and their families) who accounted for over half of all visits by relatives. Relatives were also an important source of help, for example, with the shopping (where this was needed) and providing transport.

Another indicator of social contacts with the outside community is the extent of participation in clubs and outside organisations. Approximately a fifth of respondents belonged to either an old age pensioners' lunch club, some other form of social club or a combination of these.

Support services

Respondents were asked about the services they had received in the 6 months prior to the interview. A third of tenants were getting the services of a home help at least once a week and 10% received meals on wheels. Approximately 30% had received a visit from the district nurse but this type of visit might be relatively infrequent. Almost two-thirds of tenants had seen their GP in the last 6 months. Respondents were also asked if they had received these services in their previous home and this information suggests that there has been a fairly large increase in the percentage of tenants receiving particular services (with the exception of GPs).

The extent of this change for particular services is set out in Table V.

TABLE V

(1) Services	(2) Percentage of tenants visited in previous home	(3) Percentage of tenants* visited in 6 months prior to interview	(3) - (2)
GP	76	61	− 15%
District Nurse	16	24	+ 8%
Health Visitor	8	19	+ 11%
Home help	13	34	+ 21%
Meals on wheels	3	11	+ 8%
Social workers	6	9	+ 3%
Chiropodist	13	34	+ 21%
Other services, e.g. physiotherapist	2	4	+ 2%

* Tenants who had been in sheltered housing for less than 6 months were asked about visits received only during their time in sheltered housing.

These results could be explained either by the effects of aging or by the tendency of tenants in sheltered housing to receive a higher level of services than the rest of the community. The findings of this study and the Leed's survey carried out by Butler[20] suggests that sheltered housing tenants receive a higher level of support in comparison with a sample of the general elderly population in England. Unfortunately, there is no comparable national data for Scotland but limited comparisons are possible with local studies carried out by Clackmannan[21] and the Borders.[5] A comparison of levels of use for individual services drawing on both these local studies and the OPCS survey in England[19] suggests a fairly consistent pattern of higher usage amongst the residents of sheltered schemes as set out in Table VI.

TABLE VI

Percentage of respondents who had in the last six months	Scottish Sheltered Housing study	OPCS study of elderly in England	Borders study of elderly	Clackmannan study of elderly
Visited their GP	61	43	*	*
Received a visit from a District Nurse	24	7.8	*	*
Received a visit from a Health Visitor	19	4.4	*	*
Received a visit from a home help	34	8.9	*	*
In receipt of meals on wheels	10	2.6	3	3
Received a visit from a social worker	9	3.9	*	*
Received a visit from a chiropodist	34	*	*	27

* Comparable information not available.

Respondents were generally satisfied with the amount of services and support which they received. Approximately 11% of the sample felt there were tasks which they would have liked more help with - the most frequently mentioned were bathing, shopping and housework.

Attitudes of general practitioners

A survey of general practitioners with patients in sheltered housing schemes was carried out (84 in total) as a separate part of the study. 61% of GPs thought that sheltered housing improved their ability to provide medical care for the elderly. They referred to the advantages of close supervision by and regular contact with the warden, which led to rapid notification of signs of ill-health. In addition some GPs mentioned the specific advantages of having their patients grouped together, thus cutting down travelling time and giving the GP more time with individual patients.

Attitudes of health board staff

Interviews were also carried out with 24 respondents responsible for health board staff serving schemes covered by the study. Over half these respondents thought that sheltered housing had no effect on the workload of their staff. In 3 districts an increase in work was reported as a result of the influx of elderly people into their area and because wardens increased referrals, whilst 2 districts reported a decrease mainly due to the saving in travelling time.

Despite the different effects on workloads, only 3 respondents said there had been changes in their staff organisation. In one case it had been necessary to employ more staff and another respondent mentioned an increase in the amount of time worked by the nursing auxiliaries to cope with the extra workload.

The 24 respondents were responsible for different types of staff. Some supervised health visitors while others were responsible for district nurses, state enrolled and nursing auxiliaries. They were all asked if they felt that the introduction of sheltered housing had led to a more economic use of their staff resources. In most cases sheltered housing had made little difference. However, in approximately one-third of the cases the respondents felt it permitted a more economic use of staff resources. In the two rural districts particularly it was felt that staff were used more economically through savings in travelling time.

Attitudes of social work staff

Interviews were carried out with the respondents responsible for providing services to at least one of the schemes in the sample.

The effects of sheltered housing on social work staff workloads were similar to those indicated by health staff (i.e. in some cases there was an increase [5], in some a decrease[4] and in some no change[5], again with similar explanations).

As was the case with health staff, sheltered housing was seen by a considerable proportion of respondents to lead to a more economic use of social work staff.

Links with the community

To assess the success of sheltered housing as a means of retaining elderly persons in the community requires a relatively clear definition of what 'being in the community' means in practice. A very strong test of the extent to which residents of sheltered housing schemes remain part of the community might be the extent to which elderly persons retained their previous life style and social contacts. A very weak test would be the extent to which the sheltered housing scheme had become self contained so that residents had few contacts with "outsiders" apart from professional staff. The Scottish study was not designed to assess this question in any precise way, but it is clear from the limited data obtained that some elderly households retain an active social life outside of the scheme; the majority have regular contact with their relatives and a significant minority belong to outside clubs of one sort or another. Consequently, there is a *prima facie* case that residents of sheltered housing schemes are retained in the community, at least on the 'weak' test described above.

Is sheltered housing a success?

There is no doubt that the concept of sheltered housing provides a pattern of care for the elderly which is highly successful. The tenants' housing conditions are significantly improved, their health in the GPs view can be maintained more satisfactorily. The wardens and alarm systems provide a sense of security and reassurance, the fellow tenants a sense of companionship, and contact with relatives and the community at large can readily be maintained.

In short, the quality of life of tenants in sheltered housing in enhanced in a manner which it would be difficult to exaggerate, and the tenants in sheltered housing themselves see it that way too, judging by the levels of satisfaction discovered in this study.

There remains the question of cost, which cannot be answered systematically from the data available. Nevertheless, there were two conclusions in the Scottish study which are relevant to this issue. Firstly, it seems that the residents of sheltered housing schemes receive a higher level of domiciliary services than elderly people generally. Secondly, some of the professional staff involved in managing and delivering domiciliary and health care services believed that it was more cost effective to provide these services to recipients in sheltered housing than to the elderly in general.

The evidence on this is inconclusive and a proper exercise in cost accounting in this area might well be required to provide a more definite answer to the question. However, having done this, what 'price' can be put on the undoubted improvement in the quality of life sheltered housing offers to those fortunate enough to secure it.

REFERENCES

1. Annual Report of the Registrar for Scotland, 1979.
2. Scottish Home and Health Department/Scottish Education Department. *Changing Patterns of Care.* Report on Services for the Elderly in Scotland, Edinburgh, HMSO, 1980.
3. Bosanquet, N. *Beyond Three Score and Ten,* Temple Smith/New Society, 1978.
4. Scottish Development Department. *Scottish Housing Statistics, No. 7., 3rd Quarter 1979, Table 1, p.7.*
5. Gruer, R. *The Needs of the Elderly in the Scottish Borders.* Scottish Home and Health Department, 1975.
6. Scottish Federation of Housing Associations. *Who Cares?* Figure of 40 is based on a sample of 52 sheltered housing schemes opened for at least a year. There were some 5950 applicants for an estimated annual turnover of only 143.
7. Scottish Federation of Housing Associations, ibid., p.10.
8. The official 'target' adopted by Scottish Development Department of 50 units per 1000 aged 65 and over is based on a national survey carried out nearly 20 years ago, when sheltered housing was virtually unheard of in Scotland.
9. Scottish Development Department. *Scottish Housing Statistics, No. 12,* 31st March, 1981.
10. Butler, A. *Sheltered Housing in the 1980s: Some Implications for Policy and Practice.* Paper presented to Institute of Social Welfare Conference, Nottingham, 1978.
11. Wirz, H.M. McGinn, M. & Wilson, G. *Sheltered Housing in Scotland: a Research Report.* Department of Social Administration, Edinburgh University, June 1981. An abbreviated version of the findings will be available from the Scottish Office.
12. Help the Aged. Paper in *Voluntary Housing,* 13, 8. August 1981.
13. Sumner & Smith. *Planning Local Authority Services for the Elderly,* 1969.
14. Scottish Development Department. Scottish Housing Handbook, Bulletin 3, *Housing for Old People,* 1970.
15. Scottish Development Department. Circular No. 120/1975, *Housing for the Elderly* 1975.
16. Clark, D. *Sheltered Housing for the Elderly in Scotland.* Scottish Federation of Housing Associations, 1980.

17. Boldy, D. 'A Study of the Wardens of Grouped Dwellings for the Elderly'. *Social and Economic Administration*, 10, 1, Spring 1976.
18. Butler, A. & Oldham, C. Department of Social Policy, University of Leeds. (Report not published at time of going to press).
19. Hunt, A. *The Elderly at Home: a Survey carried out on behalf of the DHSS by the Office of Population Census and Surveys*. HMSO, 1978.
20. Butler, A. & Oldham, C. 'Profile of the Sheltered Housing Tenant' in *Housing*, June, 1980.
21. Band, R. & Carstairs, V. *Services for the Elderly*, A Scottish Health Service Study - in press.

ADDITIONAL REFERENCE

Thompson, C. & West, P. 'The Public Appeal of Sheltered Housing'. *Ageing and Society*, Vol.4, Part 3, Sept. 1984, 305-26. (Using questionnaire data on preferred and projected care arrangements, idealised solutions are compared with the actual arrangements made by or for old or disabled people.)

Bereavement

Gerard Rochford

INTRODUCTION

In this article I set out the characteristic phases of the bereavement experience, give some account of the prevailing theoretical perspectives on loss and mourning and relate these perspectives to the practice of bereavement counsellors. I discuss internalised and socially reinforced taboos which prevent healthy mourning and discuss the starting of a bereavement service. This is followed by a final section describing some organisations and models of practice currently to be found in the United Kingdom.

Although throughout I have in mind an elderly person's loss through death of a spouse, it will be clear that for theoretical and practice reasons such a loss cannot be split off from other losses experienced through the life-cycle. We all lose infancy, adolescence, youth, parents, friends, lovers, hopes and the breast's security. But the loss by an elderly person of her* spouse has perhaps special poignancy for when that loss is felt it encounters all those other earlier losses. As death approaches mourning may lead either to a final sense of internal restoration or of permanent depletion. The outcome is heavily dependent on earlier experiences of loss.

THE CHARACTERISTICS OF MOURNING

The characteristics of mourning following Bowlby[1] are usually organ-

* Since the typical experience of mourning is of an elderly widow I have used the feminine pronoun throughout. I also use when referring to social workers, health visitors and home helps, professions in which the female prevails.

ised according to stages, or phases, developmentally described and consistent with those theories which relate present coping processes to early, particularly infantile, experiences. The concept of stages tends to encourage the view that progress is orderly, the stages or phases discrete and that they must all be entered and passed through 'cleanly'. Perhaps also the concept of stages encourages impatience in the family, friend, neighbour or counsellor who look for progress, and fail to capture the ambivalencc of feeling, the to-ing and fro-ing, which seems to pervade the experience of bereavement. Maybe the word 'stance' is closer to the tentativeness of the desire to move on and the fear of betrayal which pulls you back.

The stances of a bereaved person, as described by several writers[1][2][3][4][5][6][7] will include many of the following features:
Shock, numbness, dazed withdrawal; denial, disbelief, a feeling of isolation, of being in a dream, of being childlike, of detachment; overactivity or physical collapse. The funeral often marks a transition: loss of religious faith may be experienced. The funeral also take on the process of idealisation, only the good is remembered[41].

Yearning and protest, pining, weeping and anger; pangs; illusions, misperceptions, dreams and hallucinations of the lost one; psychosomatic symptoms of anxiety and fear, panic, sleeplessness, palpitations, dryness of the mouth; self-neglect. The bereaved may disbelieve and deny death, speaking as if the spouse were still alive and imminent, trying to get close, to a chair, a bed, a grave; make nostalgic journeys yet showing fear of other haunts which are now dangerous, places which were previously entered, as it were, on her husband's arm. The impulse to recover the lost one, the desire for magical restoration, may be shown in the repeated rehearsal of events leading up to the death, the 'if onlys', the calling, the accusations. There is a sense in which the desire to recover, retain, restore the lost one succeeds; for the disappointment of the search, as reality insists upon its truth, can engender in the bereaved person a more relaxed sense of internal presence. Perhaps the most disturbing feeling of all is the feeling of triumph, 'I am alive and he is dead'. There are thus disturbances of thought, feeling and perception, which are attended or followed by feelings of foolishness, shame, frustration and anger.

Despair, apathy and a feeling of emptiness or meaninglessness signal belief in the death. Bitterness, irritation and hostility to others may emerge, with, usually muted, expressions of guilt and anger. The bereaved person senses the world as a dangerous place, withdraws and becomes disorganised, aimless. There is a giving up of associations with the lost one, while retaining one chosen 'version' of him, for example a photograph.

Re-organisation and adaption follow, the bereaved person re-emerges, rebuilds social relationships, restores herself. The sense of mourning as a duty is relinquished, an act that may require the 'permission' of a trusted person. It is now possible to reminisce about happy and unhappy times, with an appropriate sense of the lost and the retained. The reality of reminiscence replaces the unreality of denial. The 'good enough' survivors replace the 'resented, intrusive' substitutes.

It is clear that there are no feelings unique to the loss through death of a loved one. The processes of denial, search and realisation, the amibivalence of feeling, the contradictions of thinking and the errors of perception are the familiar experiences of reflected consciousness as we stand amid what was, what is, what we would like and what ought to be. These processes in particular occur not only within the bereaved but within the dying and within those who, in whatever capacity, share intimately the experience of the dying and the bereaved.

THEORETICAL PERSPECTIVE

We may understand the neurotic as someone who, due to constitutional, personal and social-environmental forces got stuck within a developmental process which most people travel through. So also in bereavement some get stuck but most journey through. Theoretical understanding of bereavement draws together the reciprocating knowledge of the normal and the abnormal experience, and of adult and child experience. This perspective requires us to listen not only to carefully designed research investigations but also to the analysis of practice experience and the anecdotes of the wise. For even an anecdote, honestly told, is valid data when theory is concerned with a universal phenomenon.

The prevailing theoretical perspective is psycho-analytical, a fact of special aptness. The case which first drew Freud to his life's work was a young woman treated by Breuer, whose symptoms were in response to her father's illness and death. Freud comments: '… her symptoms … correspond to a display of mourning, and there is certainly nothing pathological in being fixated to the memory of a dead person so short a time after his decease; on the contrary it would be a normal emotional process' [7]. It was this patient who called analysis 'the talking cure' and years later Leared said of the bereaved 'All they need really is to be able to talk about what has happened, in order to give full expression to their grief' [8].

The analytical perspective has developed from Freud's *Mourning and Melancholia*[9] through Klein's *Mourning and its relationship to Manic-Depressive States*[10] to Bowlby's work on attachment and loss[11], overlapping with the continuing work of Parkes[2], which incorporates the construct of 'assumptive worlds' and social transition theory.

There is a fine and moving blend of theory, practice and personal experience in *Death and the Family* by Pincus[4] and refined expressions of mourning in *A Grief Observed* by Lewis[12], Stott's *Forgetting's No Excuse*[13] and *Grief and How to Live with It* by Morris[14].

The analytical perspective has at least three implications for those, whether family members, volunteers or professionals, who respond to the bereaved. Firstly bereaved persons cannot be understood except in the context of two resonating sets of relationship, the primary ones of their infancy and the later adult relationships particularly the marriage bond.

Secondly, bereavement through death induces a process which in its manifestation and in its internal feel is in some sense a repetition of the separation anxieties of infancy and the attendant guilt as represented in the statement 'my naughtiness drove her away'. Thirdly, an enabling offer cannot be made to a bereaved person except by reaching into our own losses, whether these be of infancy or of adulthood or both. Hence the special gifts that can be offered by those who have themselves grown from their own adult mourning, who can approach the bereaved from their own creative wounds. The proper assumption for practice has been put by Freud with nice severity - '... although grief involves grave departures from the normal attitude to life, it never occurs to us to regard it as a morbid condition and hand the mourner over to medical treatment. We rest assured that after a lapse of time it will be overcome, and we look upon any interference with it as inadvisable or even harmful' [9]. I take interference to mean anything which tends to suppress the expression of grief.

The development of bereavement services would therefore be predicated upon a simple point, unanimously made, which is that mourning is a necessary process for healthy living. This, if it is not an obvious truth, arises out of another simple point, emphasised by Winnicott, that normal happiness begins within the mother-infant dyad and is sustained later within an intimate adult pair, relating to and in turn relaying a facilitating environment[15]. Loss of the dyad is the definitive loss.

THE TABOO ON GRIEVING

We may justifiably question whether the environment, intimately and socially defined, sufficiently facilitates the normal need to grieve. The taboo may be conceptualised as operating from without as well as from within, and can be seen in psychological and sociological terms. Thus a lonely person, an isolate, may be an 'unexpressed griever', whose previous losses have disabled her from expressing later losses. The tendency to shield children from the experience of a dying parent or relative may inhibit their ability later to respond healthily to death. Wessel[16] has shown that it is possible to help children express their grief and that this should be done. Parkes[3], considering the finding by Stern et al[18] that the elderly express their grief less overtly, speculates that this may be because their grief is suppressed in the presence of younger persons who cannot cope with it. This would be part of the more generalised taboo on old age, the 'fear of contamination' which is undoubtedly implicated in the reluctance of social workers to work with the elderly even though they represent a high proportion[18] of client referrals. The worth of an old person, and therefore of their feelings, is indicated materially by the poverty in which they are forced to live[19] and spiritually by the rationalist assumption that death is the end, an assumption that has its social expression in the euthanasia movement. In social work and social policy accounting, the 'value' of an old person is low and this in turn is an expression of society's values[18]. These 'values', taboos, will find their reciprocal within the person, affecting both the expression of grief and our ability to respond to it in others, especially if they are old. The taboo can also be seen in the segregation of services for the elderly, Homes for old people, pensioniers' clubs, senior citizens' holidays and rail concessions, eventide hospitals and day centres; segregations and condescensions which have their tangible and most vicious ally in the decimation of income at pensionable age, which inevitably restricts the social participation of the elderly in the wider community. The process of isolation and loss is thus enhanced by policies which herd the elderly towards social networks, both formal and informal, which are continuously depleted by death and away from networks replenished by birth. When death occurs another manifestation of the taboo is the blocking of grief by drugs which, claims Parkes, is responsible for much of the physical and mental illness which sometimes occurs among bereaved people[3]. He also suggests that the abandonment of ritual has removed both an opportunity to mourn and a clearly signalled 'closing time' for approved mourning, which could also be seen as the permission to move on.

One way of moving on would be by remarriage. But the remarriage rate for the bereaved over 55 is very low, 3 per thousand for women and 22 per thousand for men[20]. Pincus refines the concept of taboo operating against both the elderly and the bereaved by pointing out that whereas widowers are 'made to feel precious, like eligible bachelors', widows feel rejected and avoided, 'touched by death' [4].

The taboo is also expressed in the hospitalisation of dying. The majority of our population die in hospital, mostly under sedation, away from children, friends, relatives and even spouses[21]. Dear ones are ushered out, death is rushed over[4].

The hospice movement, reaching out into the homes of the dying and the bereaved, represents a determination to normalise, desegregate, and allow significance, rather than hospitalise, shut away, divest and otherwise collude with internalised and societal taboos[22].

THEORY AND PRACTICE - APPROACHING A BEREAVED PERSON

The appropriate therapeutic stance is indicated both implicitly and explicitly by various writers. Mrs. Klein[10] says that the normal working through of mourning relates to the way in which the person first deals with this process in infancy. When the good person (mother) has gone she becomes bad and this gives rise to the ambivalence of love and hate. One way of coping with loss is by internalising the lost person, sorting the good and the bad. The paradoxical effectiveness of this process, stressed by Bowlby[11], is that the ability to tolerate separation-anxiety is a sign of deep attachment. Similarly in bereavement, deep attachment leads to a corresponding deep loss, but also to the greater likelihood of restitution, as Pincus so movingly illustrates[4]. Deep attachment leads to healthy mourning as the strength of the remembered good person is retained and drawn upon, and as emotion is withdrawn from the really dead person. This parallel process, of letting go and of harvesting, eventually allows the bereaved person to talk with equanimity about both the good and the bad.The reality of the death and the reality of memory both assert themselves. Just as the anger and hatred against the dead revive and spring from infantile feelings, so also the infantile sense that naughtiness drove the mother away can be seen in the bereaved person's guilt and sense of responsibility for the death, 'if only I'd looked after him better', 'if only I'd made him go to the doctor'. Some share of the ambivalent feelings of the bereaved towards the self and the other, will also be felt by friends, neighbours, relatives, helpers and counsellors, however well intentioned and however actually helpful. The irrationality of this may be a further source of guilt later, as the bereaved person recalls this time with some shame. Substitutes for the lost one may expect both thanks and resentment. It is Parke's[2] view that prolonged or delayed mourning is usually attributable to excessive guilt and/or pronounced ambivalence in the relationship to the deceased. Kubler-Ross[5] sees the somatic symptoms of the bereaved as a failure to work through guilt, and its attendant unconscious punishment, a view which clearly borrows from our understanding of hysteria. The starting point for Pincus was to 'explore whether ... various responses to bereavement might best be understood or even predicted by focussing on the particular relationships which made for unique family patterns'[4]. The extent to which the relationship had been enhancing or depleting, whether the one was engaged with or lost in the other, interdependent or dependent, will find expression in the extent to which losing the other is being lost oneself. The internal representation of these relationships in the survivor will determine whether or not the taking in and giving out of what was good and bad was achieved without depleting, an experience which can then be drawn upon for the work of the restoration of the self in relationship with survivors. The fact that this is rarely fully achieved is indicated by the very low re-marriage rates among the bereaved of all ages[20].

The extent of the loss is also illustrated by the finding of Young[23] that the death rate for widowers over the age of 54 during the six months following the wife's death is 40% higher than for married men of the same age sample. Three-quarters of these die from heart disease - the broken-heart syndrome.

It is clear that an enabling response to bereaved persons requires sensitive and 'risky' use of self, particularly the ability to live within ambivalence and not be tempted to 'reason' with contradictory feelings. Signposts are provided by those who have been there before and some of the notes for the journey are refreshingly practical. Counsellors should allow 2 - 3 hours for the first visit, but this should not be taken as a prescription to 'hang about'. The anniversary of the death is likely to be a particularly unsettling time. Forewarned is forearmed. During the course of mourning a counsellor can expect thanks and resentment[2]. The outside world, still stable, anonymous, unaffected, indifferent, is, for a bereaved person, a particular stimulus for anguish and meaninglessness and it is important not to try to impress reality on the sufferer. Rather strengthen changes as they appear; the realisation that interaction with the lost one is now one-sided, the emerging sense of self which is the other side of loneliness, the separation and then the relocating of the self in the social world are all feelings which can be confirmed as they emerge. Talking about the lost spouse will help to retain her sense of biography as she finds her place between what is lost and what remains[6a]. The use of scrap-books with children in care has a similar purpose. Smith[6b] particularly emphasises the importance of the social context in which the bereaved person experiences the loss. This context can either hinder or facilitate the process of recovery and should be drawn on accordingly. She also says that the crucial nature of loss lies in the essentially personal experience of the bereaved. Her approach may particularly appeal to social workers who are unskilled in the application of psycho-analytic perspectives.

STARTING A BEREAVEMENT SERVICE

For those who wish to start a bereavement service, whether individually, or as policy-makers planning a fully developed resource within statutory or voluntary agencies, the way is well trodden and there is no shortage of experienced advice, literature and training manuals. Working with established movements is the obvious first step.

Cruse aims not only to establish and support new branches but also offers to train those who work with and care for the dying and the bereaved. *The National Corporation for Care of Old People* publishes, bi-monthly, a literature search, which includes a section on *"Death and Bereavement"*. *Age Concern* has recently produced *Bereavement and the Elderly* a training aid[24]. *MIND* has published a *'Bereavement resource list'*[25], which contains lists of books, articles and useful addresses. An account of St. Christopher's bereavement service can be found in *Bereavement Visiting*[22]. A direct account of the value of volunteers can be found in *The widow as caregiver in a programme of preventive intervention*[26]. *The Scottish Citizens' Advice Bureau* has published *Practical Problems after Death*[27]. Other literature and addresses are listed at the end of this article.

It is clear that bereavement services can be confidently and most aptly developed by the use of volunteers. Such a policy decision can be taken in the knowledge that it will please the finance committee but is not taken for financial reasons. A report to Kent County Council Social Services, on social care for the terminally ill at home and the bereaved, indicates the value of small scale local initiatives[28]. For those not convinced that such a service is needed read Leared's *'Problems of bereavement: the need for counselling'*[29], which was written after the experiences of the Camden Project. Those who approach such planning and practice, in fear and trembling, will find the characteristic quality of people who work with the bereaved is hope, a quality which pervades the literature and the agencies.

So the first task in the development of services is to identify and work with and through currently existing volunteer and self-help groups. The second order of development would be the releasing of social workers, home helps and health visitors for normal bereavement work. An incentive for so doing may be found in a study carried out by Social Work Service and East Sussex Social Services Department which reported that a significant number of residents in old people's homes were admitted because of bereavement depression, admissions which home-visit counselling may well have reduced[30].

The advantage of releasing and supporting home-helps and health visitors for this work relates to continuity of contact, for they will often have been involved before the death occurred. As Kubler-Ross has shown, some of the bereavement work can be done before the actual death, particularly around feelings of guilt[5]. There are in any case real advantages in the practical and the nurturing role, being combined, as the Camdem Project discovered[3]. Psychologically viewed, the counsellor's continuity in the face of the dying and the death represents an undamaged survivor who is close enough for the bereaved person to draw hope from. The worker will also have seen, or with some support, come to see, that the phases of coming to terms with and for the dying are similar to, and at root the same as, the phases of bereavement, phases which the worker herself will have experienced.

Continuity of personal contact is of course a general issue in service provision. The experience of abandonment is common to a child placed in care, an elderly person placed in a home, a sick person moving into or out of hospital, a family and widow when the patient dies. All these are likely to be abandoned by their carers at the point of transition. Leared[8] says that the bereaved want the person who has seen them in their distress to see them through. They do not want to be referred on. There is a need here for greater flexibility in agency boundaries and roles.

There is an additional nuance to the concept of continuity. Not only should it be provided by one person, so handing over is ill-advised, but 'bringing someone along' e.g. a student in training must be handled with delicacy, for it can induce regression, be felt as intrusive, give rise to the feeling that the care is not 'for her but for the student'[4]. This is not to say that students cannot be sensitive and enabling in dying and bereavement work, to which at least two accounts would bear witness[31][32].

Some continuity is also important for the need satisfaction of the counsellor which should be acknowledged as a legitimate claim on service organisation. Nevertheless the goal is to widen trust in and hand over to the surviving family and social networks, the counsellor/therapist being a St. Christopher between the banks of the past and of the future. Thus for the counsellor, personal continuity should be sought in her personal and not in her professional relationships (the problem of closing cases). Smith [6a] particularly warns against the counsellor being taken into an intimate dyad by the client.

The home help or health visitor can often draw on not only the continuity of their presence, but on their experience of the twin processes of dying and bereavement. They are both well placed to do the work which Pincus says could prevent the development of unhealthy bereavement by preparing and being prepared for it. The health visitor has the advantage of being ready for this work in her profession but may have to carry the extra burden of being seen by the bereaved as a 'legitimate' target of anger against the medical profession for 'allowing the death to occur'. This serves to underline the importance of the front-line workers having a strong and reliable support system of those who care for the carers in the inevitable pain of the encounter.

The kind of skills, attitudes and tasks required for the 'holding hand' offer, particularly relevant during the days following the funeral are set out by Pincus[4]; listening, trust, acceptance, understanding, normalising; taking on ordinary tasks; regular communications by visits and phone calls, particularly important at week-ends; offering a presence which can be relied on and which cannot be put off by anger or suffering. A 24 hour phone service offered by St. Columba's hospice in Edinburgh received 112 calls in the first nine months[21]. With a little shifting of role perception work boundaries, social workers, health visitors and home-helps could all take on this work if policy-makers could give it more priority and provide the relevant support systems.

The development of policy will be concerned not only with personal services but with educating, and forcefully restructuring for social change, particularly in the face of the taboos. The medical services too, especially the hospital system, need to separate their legitimate functions from their collusive role within the taboo process - for example to control physical pain but to allow emotional pain. All of us hide within this taboo, defend ourselves with anaesthetised feeling, embrace the 'make-believe slumber-room' [5].

The need for a specialist service

A service for bereavement counselling should be a significant preventive measure. Consistently organised it would also provide an effective network for identifying unhealthy, stuck or pathological bereavement requiring specialist therapy. Although it was the experience of the Camden Project that very few persons required psycho-therapeutic help, this may well indicate the presence of a hidden rather than a sparse population. The project itself acknowledges that 'many are too shocked or too exhausted to put out a hand for the help offered' [8]. Many of these would no doubt be suffering beneath rather than within the depths of normal grief.

The importance of continuity and the likelihood that handing-on will be experienced as rejection would suggest that specialist therapy would be best provided by giving specialist training to those offering normal bereavement counselling. This however is almost certainly impractical and probably inappropriate. Assuming that the normal offer has already been sensitively made and that the bereaved person's searching/testing reticence has not been met by the collusive reticence of family, friends, neighbours and professionals the block is likely to be deep and rooted in earlier unreleased grief[4]. 'Many mourners can only make slow steps in re-establishing the bonds with the external world because they are struggling against the chaos inside'.

The enabling translation of inhibited feelings into conscious expression is a familiar task for psycho-therapists. The development of a specialist service would therefore require the funding of suitable candidates onto psycho-therapy courses. Our theoretical understanding of bereavement indicates that the training of choice should be psycho-analytical, by which the understanding and unblocking of grief for mourner and therapist alike would be in terms of 'earlier childhood reactions to loss and abandonment'[4]. Feigenberg[33] has indicated the delicacy of the task by emphasising the tension as well as the link that exists, between acceptance and denial. Denial is the manifestation that its opposite exists at some level. The one defends the person against the other's pain and in that very process proves what it denies. In a similar process, searching acknowledges loss. The therapist works at the point of tension, nudging acceptance above the surface, investing it with the energy stolen by denial. However Parkes[2], reminds us that therapy with the chronically bereaved may not be successful. Such people are usually socially isolated and seemingly without hope. They have usually had difficult marriages and carry their dependency into therapy thus making it interminable.

From the organisation of services viewpoint *intractable grief* presents a paradox. Having been referred for specialised treatment sufferers should be then referred back to a volunteer, a non-specialist social worker, health visitor or a home-help. Although this breaks continuity of care once again it is in keeping with Pincus' view that elderly and dependent mourners require *long, supportive contact,* not short-term bereavement-focussed therapy, not insight therapy. Such shuttling will almost surely have added to the experience of rejection. Accurate assessment is therefore important as a way of avoiding unhelpful referrals. It is the view of Volkan[34] approved by Pincus that only persons whose bereavement occupies the middle ground between normal grieving and identifiable neurotic, psycho-somatic and psychotic conditions are suitable for bereavement therapy. This may be particularly so with the elderly, whose participation in deep psycho-therapy is generally held as unlikely to succeed. As Bergman says referring to follow up studies, 'there is an especial social vulnerability accompanied by associated ill-health which makes support of elderly patients with depressive symptoms a heavy task. They need not only psychiatric help but physical care and social support'[35]. He also cites a study showing that Homes' admissions include a high representation of affective and neurotic disorders. Bereavement would probably be a main feature of such conditions. This limitation on the likely effectiveness of psycho-therapy with the elderly may well be part of the taboo process itself, as I feel sure Winifred Rushforth would agree. How many psycho-therapists *want* to work with the elderly? The source of empathy is the acknowledged self, of rejection the denied self. A powerful part of the denied self is the ageing, dying self. The blocked elderly bereaved is a victim of the general taboo surrounding grief and death, which seems to be part of the taboo on tenderness identified by Suttie[36], and of the deeper 'taboo on weakness' identified by Guntrip[37] whereby patients remain half way in and half way out of treatment. As one of his patients said "If I could feel loved, I'm sure I'd grow. Can I be sure you genuinely care for the baby in me?" Hope resides in the belief that everyone has the abiding capacity to love and be loved, if only that beginning can be reached and the self reborn. In bereavement the need to regress is expressed by the woman who felt that crying was like 'wetting her knickers'; by the woman who wrapped herself in hot, wet towels and curled up in her favourite chair 'as in her mother's womb'[4]; and by the seventy-seven year old widow who said 'You curl up in bed and feel comforted'. With one voice writers are agreed that to reach such feelings in others we must reach them in ourselves. Kubler-Ross[5], speaking of Cecily Saunders, says that since she does not need denial, she is unlikely to meet such denial in others. This is another reminder that the bereaved will be selective about who she shares her grief with. That some can never share is a reminder that as Marris[38] and Wills[39] in another context, have said, the lonely seek a particular companion and not company itself. The carer can never be a replacement. Searching, even in 'resolved' mourning, always remains[4]. For most bereaved persons regression serves to find a secure position from which to set out again. For a sad few that point of security ever recedes.

ORGANISATIONS AND MODELS OF WORKING

Cruse, founded in 1959, is a national organisation with over sixty branches over Britain. It provides bereavement counselling, pratical advice and social activities, and emphasises the ways in which the bereaved can help each other. It selects, trains and supports its own volunteers who visit the bereaved and their families at home. It draws upon other professionals as consultants and also undertakes and publishes related research.

Not only does Cruse attend to the inter-relationship of practical, material, physical and psychological problems; this is mirrored in the network of resources it draws upon, covering financial, legal and housing expertise, and continuously collating and publishing relevant information from the statutory and voluntary social services .

The Camden Project (Parkes in collaboration with Camden Council of Social Service) established a bereavement service which has spread into other boroughs and counties. The model was one in which the direct service was provided by volunteers, establishing contact first by letter and, only when the offer is clearly accepted, by visits. Visits can be daily, averaging out to once a week. The volunteers themselves are supported by professional consultants and by each other, in group meetings in which the emotional stress of such work can be shared. Volunteers are chosen for their willingness and sensitivity, the process of selection being conducted in group meetings with currently active visitors. Client referrals are self-referrals, but may come via doctors, social workers, other voluntary agencies, and also friends and relatives. Jean Leared, an original consultant to the *Camden Project* has stated her task as follows: "Voluntary workers are human beings who can sympathise with this pain. For this they do not need training. I am there not to teach them, but to provide support - to support them from becoming overwhelmed by the very passionate feelings of guilt and anger so often expressed by the bereaved".

There seems to be no doubt that bereavement counselling confirms the view that the carers themselves must be cared for and that any service will founder if that need is dismissed as an indulgence.

Another important value expressed in the *Camden Project*, was that material and spiritual help are inseparable. From the beginning the project worked with the local *Citizens' Advice Bureau*. One of the advantages of this link has been that persons who find it difficult to approach others with their grief may do so via the presentation of pratical problems.

The presenting symptom does however need to be respected. The *Manchester Family Welfare Association* ran a bereavement service having noticed the number of social work referrals precipitated by bereavement. When the bereavement service was advertised overtly referrals dried up. When they reverted to offering a 'family service' they found that once again about one-third of their clients came with troubles dating back to a death[40].

The *National Council of Social Service* set up a *Bereavement Projects Group* to act as a co-ordinating body for the different bereavement groups, the aim being to bring together all those working on bereavement projects, to discuss experiences and policy. The *Dignity in Death Alliance* brings together forty organisations representing pensioners, voluntary agencies, working with and for the elderly, as well as churches and an increasing number of those concerned with the young. Another relevant grouping is the *All Party Group for Pensioners. The Samaritians* embrace bereavement counselling as part of their general mission with distressed persons. *The National Association of Widows* offers companionship and support as well as help with financial problems.

Although this article is concerned with bereavement and not with dying, it is obvious that for spiritual, psychological and practical reasons they are inseparable. Prevailing theories of bereavement all testify to this and Feigenberg[33] has identified the following stances taken by persons facing death; denial, acceptance, hope, despair, revolt, submission, disintegration, restitution, regression, security, insecurity. The similarity to the bereavement experience is clear.

The *Hospice* movement is an affirmation of the seamless web concept of existence and its relevant caring response. In Britain, the hospice movement is strong but scattered and provides a good example of tokenism in official political response. It is praised, respected and admired. However, placed firmly within the hospital tradition, its other parent, Christianity, makes it heavily dependent on the voluntary sector for funding and for development thrust.

The hospice movement, founded by Mary Aikenhead and the Irish Sisters of Charity in the last century, has its contemporary point of reference in *St. Christopher's Hospice*, Sydenham. It is pioneering in that Dame Cecily Saunders saw clearly and mobilised the resources of family, social networks, volunteers (who do the bereavement counselling and may be former clients), inter-professional collaboration and the strengths of the dying person. The vocation is practised within and between the home and the hospice.

In Scotland, the *Macmillan Home Care Service* was set up in association with *St. Columba's Hospital*, Edinburgh (opened in December 1977), having already established homes in England, some, in Cheadle and Stoke-on-Trent, subsidised by the National Society for Cancer Relief. (It was estimated in 1977, that the capital funding for a hospice was at least £300,000). Some Macmillan houses have been taken wholly within the N.H.S. for example *Countess Mountbatten House* in Southampton. Other home care services have from the beginning operated with the N.H.S., for example, the *Macmillan Unit in Christchurch*. The insistence within the hospice movement of the relevance of the spiritual and the practical, the psychological and the physical, of faith and of skill, seems to be appropriately represented in the reality of its financial dependency upon state provision <u>and</u> individual charitable giving, however much a struggle that is.

CONCLUSION

There is distinct reluctance to engage others in one's bereavement and of others to so engage. This is in part the taboo process at work, and in part a proper standing back from people's intimacies. The many disadvantages of the hospitalisation of birth and of death should make us wary of the more aggressive intrusions of some American thanatology. It is right that bereavement services should be quiet offers, and that a counsellor's entry should be by invitation. The offers should nevertheless be firmly made, the services stable and well financed, the policy clearly stated. One particular path should be followed if social services are to facilitate people, particularly volunteers, who seek the privilege of working with the bereaved. A bereavement service should give back to ordinary families their own ordinary caring responses which unconscious social and personal forces have weakened and in some cases suppressed. It should help people to bury the bad and to protect the good 'as an eternal memory'[41].

REFERENCES

1. Bowlby, J. 'Processes in Mourning' in *Int. Journal of Psycho-analysis*, 41, 1961.
2. Parkes, C.M. *Bereavement: Studies of grief in adult life*. Penguin, 1975.
3. Parkes, C.M. 'Facing the Reality' in *Age Concern* No. 23, 1977.
4. Pincus, L. *Death and the Family*. London, Faber, 1974.
5. Kubler-Ross, E. *On Death and Dying*. London, Tavistock, 1970.

6a. Smith, C.R. 'Bereavement: the Contribution of Phenomenological and Existential Analysis to a Greater Understanding of the Problem'. *British Journal of Social Work*, 5, 1, 1975.

6b. Smith, C.R. *Social Work with the Bereaved*. London, Macmillan, 1982.

7. Freud, S. *Five Lectures on Psycho-Analysis, Lecture I*. S.E. Vol. XI, London, Hogarth, 1910.
8. Leared, J. in 'Sharing the Pain'. *Age Concern*, 23, 1977.
9. Freud, S. *Mourning and Melancholia*. S.E. Vol. XIV, 1917.
10. Klein, M. 'Mourning and its relation to manic-depressive states'. in *Contributions to Psycho-Analysis*. London, Hogarth, 1948.
11. Bowlby, J. *Attachment and Loss*. Harmondsworth, Penguin, 1975.
12. Lewis, C.S. *A Grief Observed*. London, Faber, 1961.
13. Stott, M. *Forgetting's No Excuse*. London, Faber, 1973.
14. Morris, S. *Grief and How to Live with it*. London, Allen & Unwin, 1971.
15. Winnicott, D.W. *The maturational processes and the facilitating environment*. London, Hogarth, 1965.
16. Wessel, M. 'The grieving child' in *Clinical Paediatrics, 17*[7], *1978*.
17. Stern, K., Williams, G.M. and Prados, M. 'Grief Reactions in Later Life' in *American Journal of Psychiatry*, 108, 1951.
18. DHSS *Social Service Teams: the Practitioner's View*. HMSO, London, 1978.
19. Townsend, P. *Poverty in the United Kingdom*. Harmondsworth, Penguin, 1979.
20. Registrar General Census, 1971. HMSO, London.
21. Doyle, D. (Ed.) *Terminal Care*. Edinburgh, Churchill Livingstone, 1979.
22. Dyne, G. (Ed.) *Bereavement Visiting:* An account of St. Christopher's Hospital bereavement service. King's Fund Publicity Officer, 120 Albert Street, London, NW17 NF.

23. Young, M., Benjamin, B. & Wallis, C. 'Mortality of Widowers'. in *Lancet,* (2) 1963.
24. Age Concern. *Bereavement and the Elderly.* A training aid. 1981.
25. MIND *Bereavement resource list.* 1978.
26. Silverman, P.R. 'The Widow as caregiver in a programme of preventive intervention with other widows'. *Mental Hygiene,* 54, 4, 1970.
27. Scottish Citizens' Advice Bureau. *Practical Problems after Death.*
28. Wells, K. *Social care for the terminally ill at home and the bereaved.* Kent Voluntary Service Council, Maidstone, 1980.
29. Leared, J. 'Problems of bereavement: the need for counselling'. *Social Services Quarterly,* 52,3, 1979.
30. Social Work Service and East Sussex Social Services Department. *Old People's Homes and bereavement depression.*
31. Taylor, F. *A psycho-social study of a terminal case within the hospital setting.* Dissertation. Aberdeen University Social Work Department, 1978.
32. Nisbet, J. *Caring for the bereaved.* Dissertation. Aberdeen University Social Work Department. 1978.
33. Feigenberg, L. *Terminal Care.* New York, Brunner/Mazel, 1980.
34. Volkan, V. 'Re-grief therapy'. in *Bereavement: its psycho-social aspects.* Ed. Schoenberg, B. et al. Columbia University Press, New York, 1975.
35. Bergman, K. 'Psychogeriatrics' in *Medicine:* Psychiatric Disorders, 9, 1930.
36. Suttie, I.D. *The origins of love and hate.* London, Kegan Paul, 1935.
37. Guntrip, H. *Schizoid Phenomena Object Relations and the Self.* London, Hogarth, 1968.
38. Marris, P. *Widows and their families.* London, Routledge, 1958.
39. Wills, D. *Spare the Child.* Harmondsworth, Penguin, 1971.
40. Heptinstall, D. (Ed.) 'Background: Bereavement Can't be Ignored' in *Community Care,* 316, July 3rd 1980.
41. Jaques, E. 'Social systems as a defence against persecutory and depressive anxiety' Ch. 20, in *New Directions in Psycho-Analysis.* (Eds.) Klein, M., Heimann, P. Money-Kyrle, R.E. London, Tavistock, 1955.

ADDITIONAL REFERENCES

Bowlby, J. *The Making and Breaking of Affectional Bonds.* Tavistock, London, 1979.

Marris, P. *Loss and Change.* Routledge & Kegan Paul, London, 1974.

Worden, J. William, *Grief Counselling and Grief Therapy.* (Foreward by Colin Murray Parkes) Tavistock, London, 1983.

OTHER INFORMATION

Bereavement Papers. Family Welfare Association, 501 Kingsland Road, London, 1978.
Gorer, G. *Death Grief and Mourning in Contemporary Britain.* London, Cresset, 1964.
Miller, A.J. & Acri, M.J. *Death: a bibliographical index.* The Scarecrow Press, 1977.
'Aspects of Bereavement'. *New Age,* Vol. 15, 1981.
New Literature on Old Age. National Corporation for Care of Old People. (6 per year). Section on 'Death & Bereavement'. Nuffield Lodge, Regents Park, London.
Smith, K. *Help for the Bereaved.* Duckworth, 1978.

The Compassionate Friends, c/o Mrs. Brenda Trimmer, 2 Nordon Road, Blandford, Dorset, DT11 7LT. Telephone 0258 52760.
Cruse House, 120 Sheen Road, Richmond, Surrey, TW9G UR.
The Samaritans Incorporated, 17 Uxbridge Road, Slough, SL1 1SN.
The National Association of Widows, Stafford District Voluntary Service Centre, Chell Road Stafford, ST16 2QA.

Practice in Residential Care

Barbara Firth

INTRODUCTION

Too often residential care for the elderly is seen in negative terms. It is a last resort, a last refuge and always second-best to remaining in one's own home. To some it conjures up images of bleak, cheerless places, full of frail, confused and apathetic residents who are segregated from the rest of the community and have abdicated any further responsibility for their own lives. Thus old people's homes are seen as places to stay well clear of, unless admission is inevitable.

Townsend[1], in his survey of residential institutions and Homes for the elderly in England and Wales, thought the very nature of communal care led to the disadvantages found in many Homes. He saw them as artificial communities in which smooth organisation and uniform methods of treatment necessarily restricted opportunities for self-expression and meant a departure from conditions of homeliness.

Davis[2], in her review of the growth of residential care, current practice and the central issues within it, points out that the idea of residential provision as a last resort also arises from an assumption that the prime responsibility for the care of dependants lies with their 'natural' families. Entry into care is then seen in terms of a 'breakdown' and a failure on the part of both the individual and the family. Practitioners are, therefore, exhorted to explore every other avenue and possible course of action and only in the last resort to consider admission to a Home[3].

A recent report on services for the elderly in Scotland[4] is of the opinion that:

> 'The most traumatic experience for an elderly person is the move from familiar domestic surroundings, no matter how relaxed and

welcoming a residential Home or hospital may be'.

It is assumed that people would rather not be in a Home because they are separated from all they have previously known and enjoyed.

However, Clough[5] in his participant observation study of an old people's home in Somerset feels it is facile to say that domiciliary services are, by nature, 'superior' and that it is preferable for all people at all times to remain in the community. Underlying such assumptions is an idealised model of community/family care, juxtaposed with a picture of inadequate residential care. Flew's[6] description of her experience of caring for a confused and frail elderly relative at home, presents an opposite view. What is apparent is the hard work and drudgery involved, without much recourse to professional support, help and advice.

At the same time, it is apparent that residential care often is inadequate. Martin's experience[7] of a placement in an old people's home in London highlights many areas of 'bad practice'. She felt the Home, which was something of a showpiece, was run for the staff and not for the residents. The Home was geographically isolated, so that residents were away from familiar surroundings and in design it seemed very claustrophobic - there was nothing to look at. On admission staff were given almost no information on new residents, who brought with them only their clothes. The field social worker generally severed any links at the point of admission, when cases were closed. Residents were treated like children and had little control over any part of their lives. They suffered loss of status, loss of identity and worth, and loss of privacy. The role of the Care Assistant was reduced to a series of physical achievements done at frenetic speed, allowing scant opportunity for social contacts with the residents. The Matron rejected any idea of Care Assistants each being responsible for a group of residents and also thought staff training was unneccessary. Conditions of service laid stress on the physical care of residents with almost no mention of their social and emotional well-being.

Martin's impressions are, then, very negative in that the Home seems to add nothing to the life of its residents. At the same time, it is probably inevitable that many people will require some form of residential care. Hudson[8] in his examination of those practices which make residential provision more acceptable to the elderly, points to the fact that the trend is towards more old people living alone, reflecting the greater mobility of children leaving parents. Allied to this is the anticipated increase over the next twenty-five years in the numbers of the very old. He feels that domiciliary services cannot be expected to cover all the needs of the elderly, expecially the physically frail.

An added difficulty in the provision of care and services for old people is that the providers and architects of such services have themselves never experienced old age, whereas everyone engaged in child care has had an experience of childhood. In turn, residents in Homes tend to say that everything is fine, because it is often better than they expected with memories of the work-house still uppermost. These factors thus complicate the residential task and against such a background, this article will explore current theories of residential care and existing models of old people's homes and in this context review relevant research. It aims to highlight some of the main issues facing both residents and staff and to look at some positive developments in the care of the old.

THEORIES OF RESIDENTIAL CARE

Davis[2] identifies three different stances on the potential of residential care - optimistic, pessimistic and radical. The optimists see the development of residential care as the gradual recognition of and response to a variety of human needs. It is a gradual evolution in a positive direction. They recognise that residential care is still seen as second-rate and advocate raising its status by an increase in training and clarification of principles and practices.

The pessimists, on the other hand, see residential care as static and unable to change, so that it will always be regarded as second-best provision. It can provide shelter or care when there is temporary or permanent breakdown in the basic source of care, usually the family. However, because the dominant ideology in society sets constraints on the nature of residential care, people in care are seen as rejects. There is stigma surrounding residential care which shapes the ideas and work of those involved in it.

The radicals have only recently emerged. Whilst they locate residential care in its social and economic context and see that it buttresses the status quo, they differ from the pessimists over the issue of the family. They question the assumption that residential care is inferior to life in the nuclear family. Residential care should offer a positive option and create residential solutions which do more than reflect the dominant concerns of the present political order. The problem is how not to create a unit divorced from the outside world.

Using this analysis it is possible to find a strong pessimistic trend running through discussions of residential care for the elderly. Townsend[1] in his study of old people's homes saw them very much as second best provision with little hope for improvement. There does seem, though, to be an optimistic strand emerging which, whilst critical of much current practice, does see the possibilities of change and improvement. Clough[5] in his study is attempting to show the circumstances in which living in a Home can be for certain people, the way of life they themselves would choose. The radical position is more difficult to identify, but perhaps some of the retirement communities in the United States illustrate this standpoint.

The relationship between residential care and family care is riddled with contradictions. Ann Davis shows there is a long history of expectation by the state that the family should care for its dependents and a fear that public care might undermine the natural networks of the family. From this grew the deterrent workhouse regimes. Gradually, such assumptions started to be questioned and residential care was sometimes seen as a solution to problems of inadequacy or described as part of a strategy to ease the burden of a family, thus helping it cope better. However the onus was still on the family to declare that it was not coping i.e. that it had failed.

At the same time as using notions of family life to criticise the practice and even the existence of residential care, the family has often been looked to, to provide positive models for residential establishments[9].

Davis[2] classifies residential provision in Britain into three groups, which reflect her concern with the relationship between family care and residential care. The three groupings she suggests are:

1. Family - substitute care
2. Family - alternative care
3. Family - supplement care.

1. Family - substitute care

This is defined as providing care as good as family care and aspires to model itself on ordinary family life. Such care, though, does face certain problems, Firstly, residential staff tend to have little say in the selection of new residents, even though the individual can affect the group. Secondly, many residents still have families of their won, so what part does the residential worker play in the relationship between residents and their families? Evidence suggests that residential workers develop negative attitudes towards residents' families. Thirdly, relationships within families are not always enabling. There is a danger inherent in the worker-resident relationship of infantilising the resident if the staff member takes a parenting role. Finally, families are not divorced from community networks, but entry into residential care often severs these links, either because of the location of the unit or the frailty of its residents.

2. Family - alternative care

The core assumptions of such care stress the limitations of family care and the pathological nature of some forms of family life. Within this form of care are traditional settings such as hospitals, as well as those based on alternative assumptions, such as therapeutic communities.

The problems of this approach are firstly, those concerned with developing family alternative regimes. It is often a step into the unknown, but, at the same time, previous attitudes or organisational styles need to be taken into account, as they can limit and continue to influence new regimes.

Secondly, there are problems with regard to worker and resident relationships, as there are no equivalent ideas, such as parenting, to draw on. Some units draw on the nursing model, whereas others look to the therapeutic community where attempts are made to enhance personal relationships between staff and residents.

Thirdly, there are difficulties encountered in what constitutes appropriate contact between residents and their own families. Hospitals overcome this by the use of set visiting hours.

Finally, the family-alternative model is said often to cause problems for the individual going back to rejoin the outside world. To tackle this transitional programmes based on the idea of rehabilitation have been developed, as well as long-term alternatives, such as units of communal living.

3. Family - supplement care

This is a recent development and is derived from ideas of maintaining dependant and deviant individuals in their own communities for as long as possible. Residential provision is seen as a positive resource and part of a community care programme offering specialist advice and practical assistance to families.

Such care can be grouped into three major types:

1. rehabilitation of the family as a unit, based on assumptions that the family unit is sick and in need of some education, training or therapy.
2. rehabilitation of the individual to improved social functioning and re-establishment back into the family.
3. sharing care with the family, offering a range of resources such as temporary care for an elderly person thus enabling the family to take a break.

Family - supplement care is an attempt to use residential provision in a more flexible way than has been done previously, but it does face certain problems. Firstly, as this is not 'last-resort' care there are difficulties in knowing when to refer, as well as whom to refer. Appropriateness of referral would seem to depend on detailed assessment, as well as the early involvement of residential workers in the selection of residents. This would require firmer patterns of co-operation between residential and field workers.

Secondly, engaging the family is an important part of such care, which, in turn, calls for an 'opening-up' of residential units. Residential workers and their methods will then become more 'visible' and thus they will have to cope with their effectiveness being open to question.

Thirdly, there are problems in the management of the transition of individuals from the unit back into family life. This can be complicated by such things as the effect of the residential experience or change and the family itself. This, in turn, can lead to 'silting', where such units become 'choked' with residents in need of long-term care but with nowhere suitable for them to move on to. In time a unit may lose its flexible approach and its original aims and turn into just another long-term, traditional residential setting. Family-supplement units need to be a means to an end, not an end in themselves.

To realise their full potential, family-supplement units will need to call on skills of assessment, individual counselling, family therapy, day-care, time-limited residential care and re-settlement. Such a wide range of skills will depend on establishing a team of individuals whose joint work will encompass all of them. It may be however that family-supplement care cannot reach its full potential in Britain where social service organisations have evolved from a view of residential units as a means of containing problems not intervening in them.

MODELS OF HOMES FOR THE ELDERLY

As part of the package of post-1948 reforms, Aneurin Bevin saw the end of the workhouse and the rise of the concept of the 'Home as a Hotel', where the 'master and inmate' relationship would be replaced by one more nearly approaching that of hotel manager and guest[10].

Local authorities did begin to build smaller Homes, but in his description of Homes for the elderly, Harris[11], believes that whatever their size and whatever they aspire to, they are really all the same. He sees all Homes as institutions in which opportunities for living are contracted and privacy, independence, and dignity are eroded. He therefore feels that as instruments of social policy, Homes for the elderly should be abandoned.

In contrast, Clough[5] identifies various models of old people's homes. He uses a typology developed from two variables: 1) the extent to which a resident controls his or her lifestyle and 2) different theories of ageing.

His first three types are based on an activity theory of ageing where, for ageing to be successful, replacement activities need to be found for those that have been given up through ill-health or retirement.

1. Nursing home

This is a staff-dominated unit and residents are there because they are not fit enough to manage outside. Emphasis is placed on organising activities and there is usually a fairly rigid daily routine. The residents tend to have minimal control over their life-style and they are expected to conform.

2. Therapeutic unit

Again the staff are dominant but they do provide for some resident participation. Residents are encouraged to be independant and success is seen in terms of accomplishments, with a 'blind eye' being turned to disabilities.

3. Retirement community

This is common in the USA and here residents make the decisions and the staff are regarded as employees.

The next three types are based on theories of disengagement in old age.

4. Institution

This is characterised by withdrawal from social activities by the residents who have minimal control of their life-style. There is a high degree of regimentation and unlike the Nursing Home model, activity is seen as something that confuses.

5. Hotel

Here residents are seen as people with influence and tend to be 'gentle' old people who 'fit in' and who regard the 'quiet life' as best.

6. Flatlets

This style reflects a separate living space for the residents in which they can lead a contented existence, having accepted that former roles have less significance.

The last three models have developed from a socio-environmental theory of ageing.

7. Home

Here staff acknowledge that individuals have different resources, but they also set the expectations for the group and for each resident.

8. Hostel

Here staff set the rules but then, within that framework, the residents have the freedom to select their own life-styles.

9. Supportive unit

In such a unit the residents have dominance. Even if they are physically dependant, they still play a major role in establishing their own life-style and admission to the unit is at their request.

Clough sees the analysis of Homes in this way as an important first step in looking at an appropriate style of a Home for the elderly. He does point out, though, that if maximum feasible control of one's life-style is seen as a valid goal for the elderly, then care has to be taken in how this is to be measured. It is important to differentiate between what is an inflexible regime and what is residents' choice supported by staff.

In 1977 a research study was carried out in Wales[12] in an attempt to look at the future development of old people's homes. Social services staff, all working with the elderly, were presented with eight models of possible Homes and asked to state their preference. The models were:

1. The *refuge* model providing short-term care perhaps to give relatives a break.
2. The *rehabilitation* model to provide temporary care to help the individual reach their maximum potential.
3. The *Assessment unit* model for short-term care with diagnostic facilities.
4. The *hotel* model for long or short-term care, available on demand, where the staff would do all the daily chores and residents would be free to maintain their independence and privacy.
5. The *extended family* model where people of all ages needing care would live together and where self-help and participation would be emphasised.
6. The *campus* model which would be a resource centre for the elderly with a total range of health and social facilities.
7. The *penultimate* model providing a secure, protected environment for the incapacitated elderly, but staff do not have nursing skills.
8. The *hospital* model where staff have nursing skills and can provide terminal care.

The results of the survey showed that the most poplular model was the rehabilitation unit, followed by the hospital model, whilst the least popular was the hotel model. Overall, the survey showed staff had a preference for short-stay, specialist residential care with shared decision-making. The problem is that the research questions do not seem to allow sufficiently for the possibility of different models being appropriate for different groups of the elderly with different needs e.g. what is appropriate for the fit and well would be different from what is appropriate for the frail and confused, or the terminally ill.

Three main implications for practice were highlighted from this study. Firstly, priority should be given to the development of sheltered housing units, providing a semi-secure living situation. Secondly, there is a need for the development of nursing homes for the very frail and this should be the responsibility of the National Health Service. Finally, local authorities need to experiment with a more differential use of beds in Homes and in particular to increase the number of short stay places. It should, perhaps, be noted here that these implications were based on staff preference. Little note seems to have been taken of other data such as the views of the residents themselves.

In discussing the many differing models of Homes for the elderly, mention should be made here of standards of care. How should these be defined? What characterises good or bad care? That this is a difficult variable to define is apparent when considering the whole question of the registration of private and voluntary Homes.

The 1948 National Assistance Act gave local authorities a duty to register and supervise private and voluntary Homes for the elderly. The legislation and DHSS guidelines for its implementation are vague, couched in terms such as 'reasonable standards', with no further definition of what these should be. It is left very much to individual local authorities to work out their own definitions. Turner[13] in her description of private residential provision found that unregistered Homes were not necessarily any worse than those which were registered. Also, many places have discovered a loop-hole in the law. If they call themselves a guest-house they do not have to be registered.

There is often ambivalence within local authorities; if they do close down a private Home they are creating problems for themselves in terms of present and potential users of that Home. In addition, if a local authority orders a private Home to improve its facilities it will often have to provide the money to do this.

The 1977 PSSC Report[14] suggested that the whole subject of registration and inspection of Homes be reviewed, arguing that if they are to provide good quality care, the role of the registering authority must be considerably more than a legalistic one. It must also include positive support and advice.

ADMISSION TO CARE - CRITERIA AND PROCEDURES

Why do some elderly people apply for admission to residential care and others not? How is an assessment made as to whether residential care is suitable and how are vacancies allocated?

Clough[5] found that the elderly themselves rarely initiated the referral but that often the GP was a significant influence in admission procedures. This can be explained in terms of GPs having the widest range of contact with the elderly, being used to making recommendations, and tending to have some status. In contrast, if a social worker was involved she was less likely to suggest admission to a Home. Instead, she emphasised independence, even when the struggle of daily living restricted independence. Clough suggests that, because doctors deal in ill-health, they have a more negative view of old-age. He also asks how far are major life-decisions for the elderly made on the casual recommendations of others?

The majority of commentators tend to stress the need for clearly defined criteria and procedures for admission into care. After the initial referral comes the task of assessment of the old person's suitability and need for an old people's home[15]. Both Brearley[3] in his guide to practice and Pritchard[15], a practitioner advocating increased social work involvement in this area, see this ideally as a social work task to be accomplished by building up a clear picture of the situation, involving all relevant parties and specifically considering the individual's attitude to his situation; his state of health; his physical surrounding; and his social environment. It is seen as important to explore any other possible options, such as domiciliary services[3], and always to involve the elderly person fully in any discussion. The client should be given time to make a decision and all possible information on which to base it. Unavoidable emergency admission can, however, wreak havoc with such ideas of planned intake and may lead to inappropriate long-term placements, suggesting the need for regular review of residents' progress.

A DHSS study of Homes in London[16] found that, in practice, few local authorities had clearly defined assessment procedures. Lothian, though, is an example of a local authority which does[17]. It describes its residential accommodation in terms of a service providing a group-living experience and aiming to preserve independence. Before consideration is given to residential care, domiciliary and hospital services must first be explored. Residential care is not considered suitable for people who are bedridden; doubly incontinent; continually incontinent; aggressive; mentally ill; physically very unfit; who wander; or are alcoholics whose behaviour is likely to be disruptive.

Lothian Social Work Department has written procedures for admission broken down into nine stages:

1. Allocation - to a qualified social worker.
2. Initial action - initial assessment to evaluate the situation. The residential worker may be involved at this stage.
3. Assessment - this includes completion of forms and contact with the GP.
4. Area or hospital team approved.
5. Allocation panel which the social worker should attend.
6. If allocated a place the social worker should then arrange for a pre-admission visit to the Home and for the officer-in-charge to visit the client at home.
7. After the pre-admission visit the social worker must arrange a realistic admission date.
8. The social worker must notify all involved parties and accompany the client on admission.
9. Follow-up - the resident should remain on the social worker's case-load for at least three months and the social worker must attend all reviews.

Such procedures are obviously an ideal model and may not reflect what actually happens in practice.

Allocation of vacancies can often present problems. The DHSS survey[16] found that local authorities tended to allocate vacancies not by position on the waiting list, but by the need at the time of the vacancy. Waiting lists tended to be a guide to approximate demand. Doubts were often expressed about their value and new ideas tried. Pritchard[15] feels waiting lists are only workable if they are dynamic, that is broken down into priority ranking with allocation from the highest categories, but the lower categories must be constantly reviewed so that they can move up should their circumstances change. This requires regular monitoring and assessment meetings.

The idea of a panel who allocate vacancies is fairly common. The DHSS study[16] found that more than a quarter of the London Borough operated in this way, although membership varied and there was, sometimes, confusion regarding role and function. Workable allocation procedures are dependant on sound assessment procedures. A recent study in Coventry[18] concluded that sound assessment would put an end to partisan advocay by social workers.

Preparing the client for admission is seen as being of crucial importance. It should include not only a visit to the residential establishment, but also a visit by the residential worker to the client's home[3]. The PSSC report[14] drawn up by a Working Group on residential care and setting out ideals of practice, feels that just one visit to the residential unit is insufficient as it does not afford enough time to get to know the Home. Short-term care or a trial period in the Home could be of some benefit here. It also sees as important the need for the policy and objectives of the Home to be clearly explained to the client prior to admission. A 'prospectus' for each Home is suggested, to include such things as what personal possessions can be brought into the Home. Admission itself, they advocate, should be gradual and unhurried, with existing residents and staff being prepared for the new arrival. This should include staff being furnished with some basic background information to help them understand the behaviour of the new resident.

Clough[5] found that, even if, prior to admission, a resident had been on the waiting list for a Home, when a vacancy arose it came suddenly and many felt pressurised. Obviously vacancies could not be planned, but there was often conflict between the need for high occupancy rates to keep down costs and the needs of the client to have time to make a decision. Clough also found confusion as to which personal items could be brought into the Home and often, concerned to do the right thing, they did not bring in what they really wanted. It did seem that the most satisfied residents were those who felt they had played a major role in making the decision to enter the Home.

Once admission had been effected Pritchard[15] advocates a review system for each resident as part of a programme for continued care, rehabilitation elsewhere, or return home. A review system is also a means of checking whether assessment and allocation procedures are working. He suggests, as a format for reviews, a meeting of the field social worker, the Head of the Home, relevant care staff, relatives and the resident, to be chaired by the person responsible for the allocation of vacancies in that establishment.

DAILY LIVING

It is often apparent that the same degree of choice exercised by someone in the community is unavailable to the average resident, for whom such things as meal-times or choice of food tend to be determined by routine and convenience[19]. However it should not be assumed that being in a Home simply restricts rights and freedoms. Often a move into residential care can increase the freedom of the individual, especially where living in the community has become one long struggle to cope adequately. The view of the group who drew up the 1977 PSSC Report[14] is that:

> 'all residents should have the right to lead a life which is as satisfying as possible in their own terms; to have their needs met with dignity, privacy and humanity; to participate fully, should they so wish, in decisions about arrangements for daily living; to take risks and be responsible for their own behaviour, where this does not reduce the quality of life, or safety of others; to have similar opportunities for mixing with the outside world to those who live in families; to use general community resources, if desired, such as hospital, dental and optical services, their own general practitioner, physical aids, educational services; to have access to facilities and equipment for physical education, domestic activity and occupation'.

Routines

Some routine is usually necessary in a residential unit, but it is often easy for routines to be regarded as impossible to change. Everything has to be done to fit in with the routine when the ideal would be a flexible and minimal daily routine, established in accordance with residents' wishes.

The DHSS study of Homes in London[16] found early rising was a common feature and often explained in terms of elderly people prefering to rise early. In fact, the reason was more usually that it was the responsibility of night staff to get people up and ready for breakfast. In some Homes residents were being woken at 5.30 am for breakfast at 8.30 am! The usual picture was one of frenzied activity by staff who felt under pressure to get through their time-table before their shift ended. Such hustle and bustle is hardly conducive to a tranquil start to the day!

In contrast, the study found a gentler start to the day in private and voluntary Homes, maybe because sometimes residents tended to be less frail and therefore not in need of much assistance. In all Homes bed-times were usually more flexible, but, even so, in some Homes pressure of time on over-worked care staff meant some frail residents were in bed by 4.30 pm.

Food and meal times are important parts of residential living, but it is an area in which there is often little flexibility and where routines are often for the benefit of staff rather than residents. For instance, the times of meals seldom vary and often, with the last meal of the day being between

4 and 5 pm[16] to suit the cook's shifts, they bear little resemblence to how people live in the community. Although the food is usually good, there tends to be little opportunity for choice. It is served directly to the residents who, Clough[5] found, tended to accept whatever was given. It was noticeable that meals seemed rushed, with staff near at hand to clear away and begin washing up. The DHSS study[16] found that in Homes where self-help was encouraged, meal-times were noticeably well-managed.

Despite the routine, Clough[5] saw that residents in the Home he observed were generally free to plan most of their day, but they could not decide to stay in bed all day. They were also confused as to when they could use their own rooms. These were cleaned every morning by domestic staff and some residents felt they were, therefore, not allowed to even tidy their own rooms or make their beds.

Privacy and personal possessions

Much lip-service is paid to privacy for elderly residents, but, in practice, life in a Home is often a very public one. It is not usual for residents to be able to lock the door of their own room[16] and often residents have to share a room. Clough[5] discusses this in terms of a resident losing the privacy of a base. Is a resident's base to be their own room or the whole Home? He found, in practice, most residents used the sitting-rooms as their normal living space. Does this mean, then, that they do have a right to a certain chair? In addition, public living exposes the individual in all areas. Other residents know the intimate details of one's physical and emotional state and sometimes, too, staff lack discretion.

Residents are mostly able to take a few personal possessions into the Home but often they are not allowed to take in furniture[16]. The reasons cited are lack of space and indeed many of the newer Homes have no facilities for storing furniture. Clough[5] realised that, despite being surrounded by one's own personal possessions, residents had little say in how the room was arranged, or the decor, and a resident had to be very strong-minded to be untidy!

Methods of handling money can contribute to loss of dignity and respect and to the image of the resident as dependant. The DHSS study[16] found only in 5% of local authority Homes did the majority of residents hold their own pension book. The residents' weekly allowance was often referred to as 'pocket money' and doled out at a set time in a public place.

HEALTH MATTERS

It is generally agreed necessary to ensure that Community Health Services are fully available to residents and this includes the right to retain their own GP[20]. In practice, many elderly residents have been and still are, at the mercy of the swop system. A consultant will only admit a person from residential care if, in turn, the Home will accept one of his patients. Many doctors are afraid, if they do admit a resident from a Home, the Home will refuse to have them back and thus another hospital bed will be blocked.

Davis[21] describing the effect of the swop system on practice, points out this has often prevented a person from receiving proper treatment at the right time. It must also make a resident feel vulnerable and show up the fallacy of the residential unit as 'home'. At the same time, doctors are in a dilemma. There are increasing numbers of elderly people in hospital who cannot return to their own homes, but, because they are receiving some form of care, have less priority for vacancies in residential Homes. It means that hospital patients often have little or no say into which Home they are admitted.

Davis advocates a total abandonment of the 'swop-system'. Residents should be admitted to hospital as and when necessary and their bed in the Home kept for four weeks. If it seems it will take longer than four weeks for them to recover, he advocates that, when ready for discharge, they should be allocated the first available vacancy in the Home from which they were admitted. People in hospital and in need of a residential Home should be assessed for a vacancy as if they were at home.

Confusion and incontinence are often seen by staff to cause the biggest problems in Homes. In the DHSS study[16] fitter residents were frequently said to be intolerant of the frailer ones, and to such an extent that in some Homes the very frail were cared for separately. The idea of separate Homes for the confused appealed to about 50% of staff interviewed, whereas the other 50% thought this would only worsen confusion. Many officers-in-charge mentioned that such problems could only be adequately dealt with if they had more and better calibre of staff, trained to understand and cope with such things as confusion and incontinence. With time and training, ideas like Reality Orientation could be of help to the confused resident[22]. It would also seem important for Homes to have up-to-date aids and equipment for dealing with disability and incontinence[20].

It seems a common practice for all drugs and medicine to be kept by the staff not the resident. Many local authorities actually specify this in their regulations. There are a few exceptions, mostly in the voluntary sector [16]. Clough[5] found there was a general feeling that, despite such a system, residents were receiving too much medication. A recent study [23] on patterns of prescribing hypnotics (i.e. any drug with sedative properties, intended to promote sleep) found that the prevalence of usage in residential Homes was less than that found for hospital geriatric in-patients, but greater than that reported for the elderly living in the community.

ACTIVITIES

The DHSS study[16] presents a rather depressing picture of activity, or the lack of it, in many homes. It found many examples of sitting areas with only a television for stimulation, whilst residents sat listlessly, either dozing or staring into space. Staff often complained they had too little time to engage in activities with residents, or that it was not worth-while to try as residents were too apathetic or lacking in interest. Sometimes Clough[5] noticed that staff were uncertain how far a resident should be left when sitting passively.

The activities most often seen in Homes[16] were singing, music and movement, and arts and crafts. Usually attendance was voluntary, but often residents felt pressurised into participation. In very few Homes were residents consulted about that they wanted, again the excuse being that they were too frail, too confused or too apathetic. There seemed to be most activity in those Homes where residents came in with activities which they were able to continue.

It is worth noting that the DHSS study found in many Homes, *as a matter of policy,* residents were not encouraged to help with chores on the grounds of the risk involved. The staff could be described as being somewhat over-protective.

Resident participation was not seen as a high priority, so, in turn, very few Homes in the DHSS study had any form of residents' meeting. Often, even if these were held they were regarded with scepticism and thought ineffective. The PSSC report[14] advocates such meetings as an integral part of the life of the Home. Whatever form such a meeting takes, it will need careful planning and staff support. If properly organised, it can be a forum for discussion and an opportunity both for residents to get to know one another better and to take part in the running of the Home.

Discussions on residential care frequently stress the importance of the residential unit not divorcing itself from the local community. Fears are sometimes expressed that residential care for the elderly will segregate them from the rest of society. The loss of independant action and the removal of the need for self-help can cause rapid deterioration, both mentally and physically, in relatively active old people. In practice the DHSS study found that going out by more able residents varied a great deal. In turn, few Homes had much in the way of community interest or input, such as volunteer visiting. Some officers-in-charge were against this, so that the stimulation of seeing new faces was sadly lacking.

DEPARTURES

Everyone will eventually leave the Home, so perhaps part of the residential task should be to help each resident to prepare for departure. Residents most usually leave residential care to go into hospital, to go to another Home or because of death. The PSSC Report[14] argues that, even though only a minority of residents receive short-term care, working towards discharge even if it will never be reached, is a sound principle. They feel it thus encourages residents to use their full capabilities. They suggest that more research is needed, especially into rehabilitation of the elderly and that staff need to be more aware of what help is available.

Clough[5] found a general fear of hospitals, that residents felt if they were admitted they would stay there permanently. Often the idea of hospital was used as a 'punishment' or a threat - that somehow they had done something wrong if they were sent to hospital.

The DHSS study[16] indicated, in most Homes, death was not a taboo subject and the terminally ill were, as far as possible, nursed within the Home. Although the physical aspects of death were openly discussed, Clough[5] thought fear of death was often hidden. Staff were usually more tolerant and reverant towards the dying and treated them tenderly, but residents were, generally, given no opportunity to discuss such things as the meaning of death.

STAFF ROLE, TRAINING AND MANAGEMENT

Staff working in Homes for the elderly have a confused task, which they are often left to carry out in the way they think best. Their work is physically demanding, emotionally stressful and often under-valued. It is rare to find any written statements of the task or of the objectives of the Home. In the DHSS study[16] officers-in-charge gave differing emphasis as to why they were there. Some saw their aim as providing care, shelter and comfort. Most stressed the need to provide a homely environment, whilst some saw the protective function as important and several gave priority to good nursing skills. The promotion of independence was rarely mentioned and some said that rehabilitation and the encouragement of independence were not objectives of the Home.

Ward[24] in examining current practice and theory, defines the main areas of work in the residential task as individual intervention; working with groups; involvement in the community; care-giving and administration. Looking specifically at work with the elderly, Brearley[25] argues that residential workers should have a grasp of the general needs of elderly people, as well as the specific needs which bring individuals into residential units. He suggests that satisfaction in old age is achieved by a balancing of inner needs, (emotional growth & adjustment) against external pressures (such as physical circumstances). Admission to a Home is a result of a crisis in this balance. The task of residential staff, he sees, as one of balancing the resident's need to feel safe and secure with their need to be independant. Clough[5] found staff were torn between conflicting expectations, between the belief that residents should be kept active, and the pleasure they derived from doing something for a resident.

As the role of the residential worker can be a difficult one, too often staff escape the emotional stresses by retreating into physical tasks, which proliferate and 'take over'. There has to be something lacking in a Home where staff cannot stop for a chat with residents[14]. The oft-quoted excuse is lack of time and that everything would be different if staffing levels were higher[16]. The PSSC report[14] suggests this is often not the case and that better staff deployment would improve matters.

The concept of the key-worker is seen as one way of doing this. The idea arose from a joint working party set up by BASW and RCA in 1976[26]. The key-worker, who could be either the field social worker or the residential worker, was seen as being responsible for the planning and implementation of an individual care-plan for each resident and would be accountable within the organisation for that case. There would obviously need to be adequate case records and regular reviews, but Elliot[27] points out there would also need to be a re-definition of role boundaries. It would mean residential workers encroaching into traditional field work territory and vice versa. It would also entail adequate supervision, not an established tradition in residential social work. However, the DHSS study[16] found that in those Homes where each staff member did have special responsibility for a group of residents, there was evidence that they knew the residents better and that pressure on staff was less.

The role of the officer-in-charge is important because, in dealing with residents, staff will take their lead from the Head of the Home[14]. Establishing adequate communications is essential and failure to do so can lead to tension, lack of understanding and frustration for both staff and residents. The PSSC Report stresses the importance of regular staff meetings for briefing, consultation and discussion. Such meetings will help to make staff less isolated but should not take the place of individual staff supervision. The DHSS study[16] found that the majority of Homes had no regular staff meetings, the reasons given were lack of time or they were not thought necessary.

As well as clear statements of objectives, qualifications and training are also important aspects of good residential work. Written job descriptions drawn up by staff and management and reviewed regularly can be of help. In reality, qualifications and training do not figure highly in residential work with the elderly, and this is linked to the confusion surrounding roles and tasks. The DHSS study found that only 5% of officers-in-charge interviewed did *not* have a nursing qualification. Only 5% also held a social work one. In turn, many officers-in-charge had little to say about the type of training needed, but a lot did lay stress on knowledge of basic nursing skills.

Elliot[19] feels it unsound to imply the skills of residential workers and field workers are totally separate. CCETSW, in its 1974 Policy Statement [27], also concluded that residential work shared with other forms of social work, a common knowledge base and common values and goals. Elliot[19] examines the two-tier system of training, CQSW and CSS. CSS was introduced as a less academically demanding level of training. Few residential workers are seconded onto CQSW courses and they are rightly suspicious that CSS will become the accepted training for residential workers. In time, some of the project work of CSS students could make a valuable contribution to the discussion of issues involved in residential care.

If staff in residential units are to work effectively, they need to have trust and confidence in management. The PSSC Report[14] looks at this whole question in some detail and emphasises the need for good personal relationships, based on mutual respect and trust. It advocates that support to the residential unit should include:

1. (a) 'Managerial supervision, managerial advice; contact with staff.
   (b) The supply of information to Homes about available services, aids and sources of advice, statutory matters, policies and projects.
   (c) The provision to Homes of administrative assistance if needed, including secretarial help.
   (d) The promotion of good communications within and without the Home, including the passing of information in either direction between head office staff, providing a feedback to the policy-makers and promoting communications between Homes, central administration and other agencies.
   (e) Liaison between heads of Homes and higher management and between heads of Homes and relevant departments of health or social services, training organisers, medical services etc. and between heads of different Homes in the area.
   (f) The maintenance of high standards of care by encouraging review and modification of work practice.
   (g) Liaison with the Training Officer.
2. (a) Supervision and consultation about professional practice.
   (b) Opportunities for individual discussion of problems and stresses with someone from outside the Home.
   (c) Opportunities for staff development, training or continuing education.
3. (a) Provision for interest to be taken in problems arising in the Home; for suggestions to be listened to and passed on.
   (b) Frequent personal attendance at the Home by those providing support.
   (c) Assistance at staff and resident meetings and guidance on their arrangement'.

It is important for the officer-in-charge to feel heard, so that the supporter must have access to senior management. In turn, the supporter must be easily accessible and support must be available twenty-four hours a day.

The reality is often very different and many staff feel themselves to be unsupported, highlighting the need for critical examination of existing support systems. The DHSS study[16] found vagueness and uncertainty about lines of accountability. Within local authority Homes, some officers-in-charge also expressed a lack of confidence in their Home Adviser, and often approached more senior management. The voluntary sector Homes seemed to benefit from shorter communication lines, as all the officers-in-charge were quite sure to whom they were accountable.

POSITIVE CARE AND NATURAL LIVING

Providing good, positive care for a number of elderly people with differing needs and various disabilities is a difficult, but not impossible task. Williams[28] describing her own experiences of working with old people in a residential setting believes that in caring for others, we must develop awareness of ourselves as individuals with individual desires, needs and life-style and through this become more aware of the individual needs of every elderly person receiving care. Residential workers must not impose their own standards but enable residents to fulfil their own needs and desires. The emphasis must be on positive approaches by staff who must, daily, provide new challenges for residents.

One approach to providing positive care is that of group-living, undertaken in old people's homes in Northamptonshire[29]. In the early 1970's Northamptonshire had built up a large stock of purpose-built or adapted Homes. They had a high level of facilities, almost equivalent to hotels, but still they were places in which few people chose to live. 'Quality of care' rather than 'quality of life' had been emphasised. A change of emphasis would involve, firstly, giving residents maximum choice; secondly, aiming to reduce loneliness by encouraging interaction between residents; and finally, maximising the involvement of individuals in their own self-care.

Gupta and Marston[29] found achieving a change of emphasis difficult. The lay-out of lounges, for example, with chairs side-by-side, gave opportunity or encouragement for people to talk with one another. The large groups of 40 or 50 residents also tended to inhibit personal interaction. They concluded that groups are only meaningful if they share some activity and that groups of 8 to 12 people are most effective. In addition, the majority of people entering residential care have some capacity for self-care, such as making their own beds or getting their own breakfast. So, in the first grouped Home, groups of approximately 8 people were set up, who shared a wide range of self-care activities.

Gupta and Marston showed that, although devisable, it was not necessary to use only Homes purpose-built for group-living. Traditional buildings can be adapted at minimal cost. The pattern of life in these Homes tends to be that residents get up when they wish, often making their own breakfast; they lay the tables; make their own tea and coffee; and clean their own rooms. Residents are not specially selected for these Homes, but it has been generally found that, after admission, their physical functioning improves and they become more active. In addition the acceleration of confusion is halted and the degree of confusion has been reduced. In turn, group living has led to a greater degree of interest and involvement from families and the community.

The concept of natural living described by Dunphy and Lodge[30] is not an alternative to group-living, but a broad basis for the direction of management in any old people's home. It is based on the idea that elderly people entering residential care should not have to suddenly change their life-style and it is linked to Clough's idea of self-mastery in daily living [31].

Dunphy and Lodge developed the concept of natural living in Homes in Leicestershire. They define its basic philosophy as one which puts *care* in the background and living in the foreground. They see the principles of natural living as:

1. Continuity of living - so that the resident does not have to make drastic changes in life-style. Clough[31] advocates drawing up a 24 hour schedule or map of how a person spent their time before admission.
2. Responsibility - because staff and residents live together in the Home, areas of responsibility should overlap.
3. Residents' Committees - as a forum for residents' views in the running of the Home.
4. Resident-Orientated living - daily programmes are tailored to meet residents' requirements.
5. Work - opportunities to work around the Home are encouraged.
6. Education - opportunities for education are encouraged.
7. Decision-making - responsibilities and decisions are taken by the residents themselves.
8. Identity - self-identification and esteem is encouraged by such things as the use of mirrors, personal belongings and staff addressing residents individually, by name.
9. Orientation - this is promoted by such things as clocks and calendars.
10. Expectation - this is encouraged in various ways, such as the menu, choice of food and by the notice board advertising future events.
11. Community Emphasis - the Home's place in the community needs to

be positively developed, so that it is accepted as part of the community.

12. Daily living activities - self-care of the individual and the residents as a group is encouraged.
13. Illness - residents are kept in the Home if they are ill, unless curative treatment can only be given in hospital.

Dunphy and Lodge see the philosophy of natural living as exciting and thought provoking, but recognise tht no change can occur without leadership, planning and delegation and that staff and residents must be fully involved in any changes. However the concepts would need to be tested and evaluated on the basis of several criteria, e.g. residents' satisfaction, staff satisfaction, ease of management and cost.

CONCLUSION

Practice in residential care for the elderly is a diverse and complex subject, with many differing strands. It is worth emphasising again, the difficulty in providing adequate and suitable caring environments for old people, that planners, carers and policy makers are (usually) not old themselves, so cannot draw on first-hand experiences, as can those engaged in child-care. Activity is often stressed, being active, doing things, is seen as the ideal - but is it? Or is it just the opinions of a younger age-group who do not appreciate the subtle changes in emphasis which take place with ageing? Activity and the maintenance of independence can, sometimes, become a tyranny, if disabilities and poor health make an individual unequal to the struggle.

Is it possible to define good and bad care? The PSSC Report[16] pinpoints some examples of bad practice such as identifying each resident with a group not as an individual; pressures to conform to expectations and routines; attitudes which diminish the status of residents in their own or each other's eyes; and lack of recognition of a person's previous skill, knowledge and relationships; over-protective attitudes; pressures on residents to conceal emotions; and finally the lack of privacy and the loss of personal possessions. Essential components of good residential care are defined as respect for privacy; encouragement to independence; availability of choice; stimulation; the recognition of emotional needs; and the opportunity to participate in organising the pattern of life.

A common theme running throughout much of the recent literature on residential care for the elderly, is that good care enables the individual, however frail, to choose as far as possible how they wish to live. It is the natural living described by Dunphy and Lodge[30]. Clough's[5] definition is a clear explanation of this approach. The prime function of the Home should be:

> 'to provide a living base in which basic physical needs are met in a way which allows the individual maximum potential for achieving mastery'.

What is the future of residential care for the elderly, beset as it is by images of oppressive institutions to be avoided unless there are no alternatives? There seems to be a strong body of opinion for contracting the residential sector and giving priority to such things as the development of sheltered housing. If this was to happen it is probable that only the frailest or most highly dependent would enter care. This could alter the residential task and residential care could become very stigmatising - definitely the last resort for the hard-core of difficult individuals. There are, though, more positive developments along the lines of Davis'[2] family-supplement care and the urging of local authorities to experiment with a differential use of beds[12].

Whatever direction residential care for the elderly takes, it is obvious there is need to reconsider and state clearly the principles and objectives of the care already being provided. For the most part, the role of staff is a confused one, thus detracting from the residential task. An explicit statement of aims and policy would enable staff to be clearer as to their function, so that quality of care, and life for residents would only improve. At the same time, staff must also be assured of strong and continuous support if they are to maintain a high level of practice. Future research might, perhaps, concentrate on definitions of the residential task and the role and place of residential Homes in the range of resources available for the elderly. Perhaps most important of all is the necessity for a closer look at the needs and wishes of the elderly themselves and how these can best be met.

REFERENCES

1. Townsend, P. *The Last Refuge*, Routledge, 1964.
2. Davis, A. *The Residential Solution*, Tavistock, 1981.
3. Brearley, P. 'Old People in Care' *Community Care Guide to Practice Supplement*, 1976.
4. *Changing Patterns of Care*, Services for the Elderly in Scotland, HMSO, 1980.
5. Clough, R. *Old Age Homes*. Allen & Unwin, 1981.
6. Flew, A. 'Looking after Granny: The Reality of Community Care' in *New Society*, 9:10:80.
7. Martin, P. 'I only came for the Flower Show' in *Social Work Today*, 9, 39, 13:6:78.

8. Hudson, B. 'The Inevitable Provision' in *Community Care,* 13:7:77.
9. Younghusband, E. *Social Work in Britain 1950 - 1975.* Allen & Unwin, 1978.
10. Report of the Ministry of Health for the Year ended 1949. HMSO, 1950.
11. Harris, H. 'Workhouse? Hotel? - it's just the bleedin' same' in *Social Work Today,* 9, 10, 1:11:77.
12. Jones, G. 'Future Models for Old People's Homes' in *Social Work Today,* 11, 9, 30:10:79.
13. Turner, J. 'The Last Refuge, where all too many people go to die' in *New Society, 25:1:79.*
14. Personal Social Services Council. *Residential Care Reviewed* incorporating *Daily Living: Questions for Staff* (PSSC 1977).
15. Pritchard, S. 'Admissions Don't Stop at the Door' in *Community Care,* 6:3:80.
16. D.H.S.S. *Residential Care for the Elderly in London.* Social Work Service, London Region, 1979.
17. Lothian Social Work Department. *Written Criteria for Admission* and *Planned Admission Procedure,* 1980.
18. Carter, K. & Evans, T.N. 'Intentions and Achievements in Admissions of the Elderly to Residential Care' in *Clearing House for Local Authority Social Services Research,* University of Birmingham, 9, 1978.
19. Elliot, D. 'Some Current Issues in Residential Work: Implications for the Social Work Task' in Walton, R.G. & Elliot, D. (Eds.) *Residential Care,* Pergamon Press, 1980.
20. DHSS Circular *Residential Accommodation for the Elderly - Arrangements for Health Care,* 1976.
21. Davies, M. 'Swopping the Old Around' in *Community Care,* 18:10:79.
22. Hanley, I.G., McGuire, R.J. & Boyd, W.D. 'Reality Orientation and Dementia: A Controlled Trial of Two Approaches' in *British Journal of Psychiatry,* 1981, 131, 10 - 14.
23. Morgan, K. & Gilleard, C.J. 'Patterns of Hypnotic Prescribing and Usage in Residential Homes for the Elderly' in *Neuropharmacology,* 20:12:81.
24. Ward, L. 'The Social Work Task in Residential Care' in Walton, R.G. and Elliot, D. (Eds.) *Residential Care.* Pergamon Press, 1980.
25. Brearley, C.P. *Residential Work with the Elderly.* Routledge & Kegan Paul, 1977.
26. BASW & RCA 'The Relationship Between Field and Residential Work' published simultaneously in *Social Work Today* and *Residential Social Work,* September, 1976.
27. CCETSW Paper III *Residential Work is a Part of Social Work,* 1974.
28. Williams, D. 'Positive Care for the Elderly' in Walton, R.G. and Elliot, D. (Eds.) *Residential Care.* Pergamon Press, 1980.
29. Marston, N. & Gupta H. 'Interesting the Old' in *Community Care,* 16:11:77.
30. Dunphy, R. & Lodge, B. 'Promoting Natural Living in a Residential Home for Elderly People' in *Choosing How to Live: Alternative Life-styles in Residential Care for Elderly People.* MIND, 1980.
31. Clough, R. 'In Residence - Mastery of Daily Living' in *Social Work Today,* 10, 13, 21:11:78.

ADDITIONAL REFERENCES

Booth, T. & Berry, S. 'An Overdose of Care'. *Community Care,* 26/7/84. (Research into dependency in residential homes.)

Davis, L. *Residential Care: A Community Resource.* Heinemann, London, 1982.

Davis, L. 'In Residence: Loneliness is . . . '. *Social Work Today,* Vol.15, No.45, 23/7/84.

Goldberg, E.M. & Connelly, N. *The Effectiveness of Social Care for the Elderly: An Overview of Recent and Current Evaluative Research*. Policy Studies Institute, Heinemann, London, 1983.

Gupta, J. 'In Residence: All Together Now'. *Social Work Today*, Vol.14, No.43, 19/7/83.

Howes, J. 'Creating a Forum'. *Community Care*, 21/4/83. (How residents of OP Homes were given a chance to voice their opinions.)

Murray, N. 'Privates on Parade'. *Community Care*, 8/3/84.

Payne, C. & Douglas, R. 'In Residence: Great Expectations'. *Social Work Today*, Vol.14, No.30, 12/4/83.

Quantrell, D. 'Life Tonic'. *Social Work Today*, Vol.14, No.27, 15/3/83.

Saxby, P. & Jeffery, D. 'In a Strange Land'. *Social Work Today*, Vol.15, No.1, 6/9/83.

Practice in Field Care

Cherry Rowlings

INTRODUCTION

This paper is in two parts. The first is concerned with the definition and assessment of need, both by professionals and by elderly people themselves. The second part focuses on some recent studies of families caring for an elderly relative suffering from senile dementia and discusses some of the ways in which 'caring for the carers' might become a reality. Wherever possible, the paper has drawn upon studies which are or have been based in Scotland.

A recent publication from the Study Commission on the family[1] makes a clear statement on the significance for Britain of an increasing number of elderly people in the population: 'expenditure on health and personal social services is seven times higher for a person over seventy-five than for a person of working age... An estimated one-third of all expenditure on social programmes goes on the elderly' (p. 64). A report from Grampian Social Work Department[2] described in more local terms the impact of an ageing population upon the region's health and social services provision (para. 1.6). 'Already half of the Social Work Department revenue budget is spent on care of the elderly. Half of all Grampian Health Board's beds and 75% of the work of district nurses are devoted to care of people aged 65 and over'. Furthermore, as the report acknowledged, in many areas resources were inadequate to meet need and the level of provision was below recommended guidelines. In this respect, Grampian will be little different from other regions nor indeed from other parts of Britain.

At team level, the implications are no less significant. If referrals are divided into the pre-Kilbrandon/Seebohm categories of elderly and handicapped, mental health and handicap and children, then those on old people form the largest group. In 'Seatown' in England, almost one-third of all referrals to the intake team in 1977 were for problems concerned with old age and disability.[3]

Figures for February 1979 from Aberdeen City[2] showed that the proportion was somewhat higher - almost one half. The ways in which referrals on elderly people come to social work departments and the response that is made makes interesting reading.

CHARACTERISTICS OF ELDERLY PEOPLE REFERRED TO SOCIAL WORK DEPARTMENTS

Apart from the fact that they are referred in high numbers relative to other sections of the community, elderly people have several other characteristics as a client group. The picture that emerged from Aberdeen[2] in 1979 was similar to that found in area teams elsewhere[3]: the majority of referrals concerned people over 70, who lived alone and who were experiencing difficulty in aspects of daily living. Hence referrals for aids, sheltered housing or home help predominated. Most referrals came from medical staff, particularly from district nurses and health visitors. Self referrals were rare. The Grampian researchers made particular comment on the form that referrals took (p. 9):

> 'A striking feature of most of the referrals ... was that a single specific service was requested, rather than presenting problems being described ... The impression gained was that the referring agent had already assessed the elderly person's needs and decided what services were required and subsequently contacted the Social Work Department in order to have the appropriate service put into operation. Of over 100 elderly people referred ... only four were referred for assessment or because of general concern about their ability to cope'.

SOME IMPLICATIONS OF ALLOCATION

An immediate consequence of this specificity of referral was that allocation was made not on the basis of the problems experienced by the old person (which were often barely mentioned on the referral form) but according to the perceived solution. Thus requests for aids went to occupational therapists, for home help to the home help organiser and for residential and day care or for sheltered housing to social workers. This is, of course, a not uncommon way of dividing up in-coming work, but relying mainly on the criterion of solution rather than of the nature and extent of the problem(s) being experienced had important repercussions. To begin with, referral agents will be guided, to a lesser or greater extent, by *their* knowledge of what resources the social work department may have at its disposal. The reliability and accuracy of this knowledge may vary. Stanley and Lutz[4] in their study of the meals-on-wheels service in Scotland commented (p. 66) that reliance upon doctors and district nurses as the assessors of need for a meals service was 'suspect'. Much depended on personal attitudes, on individual interpretations of the value of a meals service and on knowledge of the availability, or otherwise, of the service. That referral agents may not refer because they believe the chances of a successful outcome are slim is a further factor which may, in the long term, affect plans for future levels of provision. Stanley and Lutz (p. 68) sum up the problems thus:

> 'The crux of the matter, at both national and local levels, is the effect of personal perception of need on both current and planned provision. Inevitably values and attitudes will differ not only between the individuals who provide services but also between them and their clients. Discrepancies in value judgements will influence both the quality and the quantity of provision and its acceptability to the potential recipient. The data from this study highlight the differences in value judgements relating to estimated need'.

These observations were made about professional staff outside the social work department who were acting as the link men between potential clients and the services which might be of help to them. Home help organisers, occupational therapists and social workers perform a no less vital linking role; they are 'gatekeepers' to resources in their own departments and may also have some influence on gatekeepers in, for example, housing departments, social security local offices and local or national charitable organisations. Thus, the number and type of questions they ask, the manner in which they ask them and, of no less importance, the way in which they introduce the subject of alternative forms of help will affect both the level and the type of service offered to and then accepted by the client.

ASSESSMENT

The Grampian study[2] throws some interesting light on the assessment of home help organisers, occupational therapists and social workers.

Home help organisers provided the most rapid response to referral and their assessment interview generally lasted for about fifteen minutes. The immediate needs of the client were seen (p. 18) 'almost exclusively' in terms of whether or not home help services were required. (It should be said that home help staff conducted regular interviews of recipients of the service and so had the opportunity to identify further problems at a later date). Occupational therapy assessments generally took at least half an hour and sometimes over an hour. Only four of the twenty four clients were seen as having immediate needs other than aids or adaptions. The social worker assessments proved the most diverse. Individual workers varied in the extent to which they used the referral for a specific resource as the reason for undertaking a more general assessment of the client's circumstances and possible needs. By contrast to the occupational therapy and home help assessments, social workers found that their assessment of immediate need agreed with the reason for referral in only one quarter of their cases.

As with so much research, these findings generate further questions. One is whether the need for aids and for home help is more accurately perceived by referral agents than needs for sheltered housing, residential or day care. The research on the meals service mentioned above[4] suggests that we should be cautious of accepting this answer too readily. A second question is: do home help organisers and occupational therapists conduct a more focussed interview directed towards their own area of expertise and resources than (some) social workers who range more widely? Here, it must also be remembered that, whatever the diversity in length or content of interview between social work and non social work staff, there was clearly a good deal of variation *between* social workers. Indeed, the researchers commented on the difficulty of describing a 'typical' social work assessment. The different approaches to assessment of initial referrals has been noted with reference to the role of those undertaking 'duty' in area teams.[5] At one end of the spectrum were those whose unterpretation of duty was to respond to the problem as outlined by the client/referral agent and to 'clear the decks'; at the other end were those who believed in getting beyond the 'presenting problem' and in in undertaking a 'thorough assessment' of the client's circumstances. Whilst it is appropriate for individual workers to excercise some discretion in respect of how they respond to clients and problems, too much discretion may result in an unacceptable variation in service, dependent on the chance element of which type of worker 'happens' to receive the case. Elsewhere, this author[6] has argued that there should be a greater uniformity in assessment amongst the different staff in social work/social services departments who are engaged in assessing referrals on old people; furthermore, workers may need to adopt a more directive (but no less sensitive) style of interviewing, where the onus is on the worker to seek need across a broad spectrum rather than to concentrate mostly on those areas of need mentioned by the client or by the referral agent.

NEED

Studies of the elderly population demonstrate the extent of disadvantage which elderly people as a group experience. It is evident that those aged over 75 are the most disadvantaged. Hunt's survey[7] of elderly people in the community in England describes how the oldest tend to be the poorest, with an income close to the supplementary benefit level. Very old people are most likely to occupy very old houses, with consequent poor sanitation and insulation. By virtue of their longevity, they are also most likely to be alone, to receive few visits and to have outlived their family, spouse, friends and sometimes even their children.

The significance of these factors is considerable. For example, Gruer[8] found that, in her sample of elderly people in the Borders, inadequate housing was 'strongly associated' with anxiety and depression (as diagnosed by a clinician). Furthermore, over 50% of those who were socially isolated had a marked degree of depression, compared with only 8% of the non-isolated. The prevalence of depression in the elderly population is often overlooked; attention tends to be focused on the problem of dementia and indeed, depression may be misdiagnosed as dementia. But an estimated 12% of the elderly population is clinically depressed and probably nearly one-third of all successful suicides are by elderly people.[9]

The combination of extreme age, very low income (as defined by the supplementary benefit level) and social isolation were found to be significant factors in Wicks'[10] study of the incidence of hypothermia in the elderly population.

The research by Isaacs & Neville[11] in the west of Scotland showed that social rather than medical factors determined which old people entered hospital: beds were used 'preferentially for those who lived alone and who had no close relative'! Thus one sees the impact of social factors upon the well-being of old people.

Isaacs & Neville's study is one of several concerned with need in the elderly population - how it is or might be defined, how it is articulated and how far it is met. The extent of unreported need for either health or social services shows that to rely on self reporting by elderly people is an ineffective means of ensuring that services reach those who require them. Nor, as Isaacs & Neville found, can it be assumed that if an old person lives with someone else, adequate care will be available.

Studies of unreported need rely on assessments by professionals; in other words, they apply a standard of 'normative' need[12], based on expert knowledge and assessment. In their assessment of need, Isaacs & Neville[11] focussed on 'activities necessary for the maintenance of basic care' which they defined as the provision of 'food, warmth, cleanliness and security'. As the authors explained, this concern with basic care and with an individual's functional ability (as opposed to inclination) to provide these for him/herself misses out other dimensions of need - for example, the need for respect and dignity. But what it does offer is a framework for analysing the needs of physically and/or mentally dependent old people, for examining the help that is provided and for highlighting the 'fit' between the two. As a measure of severity, Isaacs & Neville used 'the interval which elapsed between necessary episodes of help'. Thus, a person who cannot do housework or shopping may be said to have 'long interval' need since help can be provided at different and varying times, and sometimes less frequently than once a day. Inability to cook or to make a hot drink comes into the 'short interval' category, since these tasks must be carried out every day, every few hours. The most serious level - 'critical interval' - includes people whose needs arise at 'short and unpredictable intervals' so that the constant presence of a helper is necessary. People suffering from incontinence, who cannot walk to the lavatory unaided, or who are severely mentally impaired may be said to have 'critical interval' need.

This method of classification would seem to be of immediate relevance to policy makers and practitioners. For example, if home help organisers were routinely to analyse new referrals in this way, important information would be made available on the level of need (*basic* need) which is present in their caseload. These categories could also be used in the assessment of old people for residential care.

Crosbie[13] and Chapman[14] have both examined the gap between subjective or 'felt' need (i.e. the recognition by the individual concerned that he/she is in need) and 'expressed' need or demand. Crosbie has suggested that there are four stages in the expression of need. First, the individual recognises that something is wrong, that he is in a state of 'dis-ease'; secondly, he judges that something should be done to correct the situation; thirdly, he has to have the knowledge that something *can* be done and finally he has to decide that he will take some action. It may be felt that, having gone through the first three stages, the individual chooses not to take action, perhaps because he is insufficiently inconvenienced to make the effort worthwhile (what Chapman refers to as 'low intensity of need'). Or the individual may be deterred from seeking help because the application procedure is too complicated or receipt of help or services is regarded as stigmatising. Chapman concluded that unexpressed need was largely attributable to lack of knowledge of the services that were available; in other words, to return to Crosbie's analysis of process, old people were 'opting out' at the third stage. This would fit with evidence from the studies on unreported ill-health amongst the elderly population, where lack of knowledge that treatment or a cure is available is one explanation why self referral to medical services is low.

REACHING OLD PEOPLE IN NEED

Chapman[14] rejects a 'blanket system of routine visiting' on the grounds that it would be 'an overreaction to a problem ... which we suggest is caused largely by the lack of good sensitive publicity for services'. He favours instead extensive and comprehensive publicity - through wider use of the media and through regular mailing lists about available services and benefits. No doubt many authorities could publicise their services more widely (although they may not wish to do so at a time of decreasing availability) but the rate of take up of social security benefits suggests that *despite* publicity, people who are eligible still remain ignorant or do not apply for other reasons. It seems questionable whether the very old, in particular, who may well be socially isolated and frail, will be responsive to impersonal contact.

Gruer[8] discussed the merits of comprehensive visiting, perhaps by a health visitor; such screening has been shown to be a successful means of identifying unreported ill-health and there is clearly potential to reveal unmet social/emotional needs through the inclusion of appropriate questions. Comprehensive visiting in the Borders, she suggested, would occupy almost 18 fulltime health visitors (an increase of 119% over current staffing levels). Screening only those aged over 75 would require less staff (an increase of 51% in establishment) but - and this is important - would uncover probably only half the unmet need. Nor would screening the known 'at risk' groups (such as those living alone or recently bereaved) be a more effective way of detecting unmet need. The message from Gruer seem clear - comprehensive detection of unmet need requires comprehensive visiting. It also has implications for the level of additional medical, paramedical and social services; as she says (p. 111) 'extra manpower needs are likely to be high' both to follow up initial referrals for investigation/assessment and also to provide a level of recurring help. Her conclusion (p. 135) is one with which few people concerned about the circumstances of many old people would disagree:

> 'The greatest need in the elderly population is money ... for individual elderly people ... (and) for the statutory services of the area'.

One Scottish scheme, *Highland Helpcall* is a system which allows elderly and disabled people anywhere in the Highland Region to call for help at any time in their own home. In case of illness, a fall, or any other emergency, appropriate assistance can be summoned at the touch of a switch on a device worn by the user. It is not necessary that the person be able to reach the telephone or even speak, and the people who answer the alarm call will in most cases be members of the person's local community. Many elderly people are very independent but they are often fearful of what might happen if they feel ill whilst alone. Such a 24 hour alarm system allows people to stay in their own home whilst giving them the reassurance that help is at hand should the need arise. Highland Helpcall also reduces the need to transfer people to sheltered housing, homes or hospital*

FAMILY CARE, DEMENTIA AND CARING FOR THE CARERS

The second part of this paper considers care of elderly people suffering from dementia, and focuses particularly on those for whom most (and sometimes all) the care is provided by their families. The contribution of the family to the care of dependent old people - indeed of dependent people of any age - has been demonstrated in a succession of studies over the previous ten years. 'Community care', in practice, usually means *family* care[15][11][16], and that, in turn, usually means care by women, or often one woman[17][18]. Isaacs & Neville's[11] use of the word 'defeated' to describe some dependent elderly people and their carers is an appropriate reminder of the cumulative effort of the struggle to cope

* Further details of the scheme are available from the Department of Social Work Highland Regional Council, Inverness. The scheme is being monitored and evaluated by Dr. Sewell of Aberdeen University.

with successive and multiple difficulties.

Gilhooly's[19] interim report on her study of family care of demented elderly people attending day hospital in Aberdeen sheds interesting light on caring and coping. It was, for example, striking that only three of the thirty four supporters interviewed gave 'senile dementia' in response to the question 'What is wrong'? One quarter said they did not know. Moreover, a significant number of respondents seemed unaware of the medical causation of dementia, attributing it perhaps to an event many years prior to the signs of dementia or expressing surprise that the demented person should be thus afflicted since she had always led a 'good' life.

Somewhat unexpectedly, Gilhooly did not find that a greater degree of impairment in the elderly person was associated with lower morale of the carer. She suggests that this may in part be due to a time factor - that at the early stages of dementia, the carer has had less opportunity to adapt and adjust to the changing circumstances. However, she is more inclined to believe that in the early stages, the carer is less certain whether the demented person really is ill or whether the difficult behaviour is wilful or deliberate. She continues (p. 9) 'furthermore, when the patient still has considerable contact with reality it is harder for the supporter to ignore the patient'. Ignoring the dementing relative was a coping mechanism described by a number of carers - leaving the room when things got too much, or going out of the house. As Gilhooly observes, if this is how many carers cope, it might be expecting too much of them to become engaged in therapies such as Reality Orientation which are designed to bring the demented person more into contact with his/her environment. Wheatley[20] describes similar coping mechanisms of ignoring and also of shouting and talking to relieve tension; her research also contributes to our understanding of the strains involved in caring. She found, as had Sanford[21] in an earlier study, that faecal incontinence caused particular distress to carers and that, where an incontinence laundry service was available, this resource was much appreciated. Physical exhaustion and loss of sleep were constant features of many carers' lives, as was a very restricted social life. The physical and emotional costs of caring are indeed great.

The need for periods of relief from caring is often mentioned by carers. Wheatley stressed that such relief must be *regular;* an annual short-term 'holiday' admission is for many carers grossly inadequate. The idea of a 'granny sitting' service is suggested by carers in both Wheatley's and Sanford's studies and Wheatley sees this as a valuable role for volunteers. However, given the often difficult task of caring for a demented person, any scheme of this nature is likely to require considerable back-up support and possibly also some form of training from social work departments. Here, lessons from the Kent Community Care Project[22] may be valuable. The deployment of volunteers, paid a nominal sum for the task(s), appears to have had success, but the social worker had a vital and central role in defining the task(s) in conjunction with both client and volunteer and then in maintaining and supporting the 'contract' between client and volunteer. Most of the clients seem to have been dependent for physical rather than mental reasons. They wanted to work with the volunteer. If social work assessment and involvement has been so important when the client was motivated to participate, it could be far more importantly - indeed essential - where the client is in many ways less engaged and maybe even suspicious, hostile or aggressive. The rewards for volunteers when 'granny sitting' with demented old poeple may be far less obvious and thus the support from social workers may be all the more necessary.

Apart from relief through possible 'granny sitters', carers have valued other forms of support. One, noted by Wheatley[20] and again in a paper presented to the British Gerontological Society at their conference in Aberdeen[23] is the provision of day care, either in a residential setting or in a day hospital. The other is the opportunity to express the experience of caring - either to a social worker[20] or to a group of carers facing similar stresses and rewards[24]. The use of support groups for carers is established in respect of, for example, relatives of schizophrenic patients or of stroke patients. Accounts by carers of what is involved in looking after a dementing relative or spouse demonstrate the need for opportunities to share experience and to compare methods of dealing with problems such as wandering. The social isolation of carers suggests that without co-ordination from outside, opportunities for meeting, comparing and supporting are minimal. This co-ordination could be appropriately undertaken by social workers, although psychologists and psychiatric nurses, to take but two other occupational groups, might see that they also could or should have a role here. There is much potential for creative teamwork in this aspect of work.

CONCLUSION

There are no neat and tidy conclusions to be drawn from the research reviewed here - except perhaps that, as Gruer[8] states, 'the estimated amount of unrecognised and unmet need, both medical and social, is daunting'. This is not encouraging reading at a time of constraints on public expenditure. But it is important that in acknowledging the situation we are not immobilised by its immensity. Moreover, a few of the possible remedies lie largely within our control: for example, the development of greater consistency in assessment between social workers, home help organisers and occupational therapists. For social workers, there is still a long way to go in understanding the *process* of work with old people; it is to be hoped that research currently being undertaken by the National Institute for Social Work will contribute to our knowledge.

For social workers, there is still a long way to go in understanding the *process* of work with old people. Here, however, research undertaken at the National Institute for Social Work throws some light on the multiplicity of roles and the extensive and sensitive work which is undertaken with and on behalf of elderly clients (25). Much of the work centred on the difficult issue of whether or not clients should remain in their current accommodation or move to an apparently 'safer' setting and there were often conflicting opinions among those involved.

A second study by the National Institute (26) provides a powerful account of the effect of caring for a dementing relative. There is a great need for social workers to become more involved and expert in supporting carers and the researchers offer useful guidelines for practice – such as the importance of informing relatives of what help is available. Many do not ask because they do not know a service exists. As social workers become more directly concerned with maintaining in the community old people who are physically and/or mentally very frail, so the challenging nature of practice with and on behalf of elderly people should become more evident.

REFERENCES

1. Rimmer, L. *Families in Focus*. London, Study Commission on the Family. 1981.
2. Grampian Social Work Department, *A Study of the referral of elderly clients in Aberdeen City* . Aberdeen Grampian Social Work Department. 1980.
3. Goldberg, E.M. & Warburton, R.W. *Ends and Means in Social Work*. London, Allen & Unwin, 1979.
4. Stanley, G. & Lutz, W. *Meals Services for the Elderly in Scotland*. Scottish Home and Health Deaprtment, 1976.
5. DHSS *Social Service Teams. The Practitioners View*, London HMSO, 1978.
6. Rowlings, C. *Social Work with Elderly People*. London, Allen & Unwin, 1981.
7. Hunt, A. *The Elderly at Home: a study of people aged sixty-five and over living in the community in England in* 1976. Office of Population Censuses and Surveys, London, HMSO, 1978.
8. Gruer, R. *Needs of the Elderly in the Scottish Borders*, Scottish Home and Health Department, 1975.

9. Shulman, K. 'Suicide and parasuicide in old age: a review', *Age and Ageing*, 7, pp 201-9, 1980.
10. Wicks, M. *Old and Cold: Hypothermia and Social Policy*, London, Heinemann, 1978.
11. Isaacs, B. & Neville, Y. *The Measurement of Need in Old People*. Scottish Health Service Studies No. 34. Edinburgh, Scottish Home and Health Department, 1976.
12. Bradshaw, J. 'A Taxonomy of Social Need' in *Problems and Progress in Medical Care*. London, Oxford University Press for Nuffield Provincial Hospitals Trust, 1972.
13. Crosbie, D. 'The concept of need - an analytical model' in Butcher, H. & Crosbie, D. *Pensioned Off - A Study of the Needs of the Elderly People in Cleator Moor*, York, University of York, 1977.
14. Chapman, P. 'Unmet Needs and the Delivery of Care'. Occasional Papers in Social Administration No. 61, Social Administration Research Trust, 1979.
15. Isaacs, B. 'Geriatric patients: do their families care'? *British Medical Journal*, 4, 1971, pp. 282-6.
16. Moroney, R.M. *The Family and the State: Considerations for Social Policy*, London, Longman, 1976.
17. Butcher, H. & Crosbie, D. *Pensioned Off - a study of the needs of elderly people in Cleator Moor*. University of York, 1977.
18. Finch, J. & Groves, D. 'Community Care and the Family: a case for equal opportunities', *Journal of Social Policy*, 9, 4, 1980.
19. Gilhooly, L.M. (forthcoming): 'The Social Dimensions of Senile Dementia' in Taylor, R. & Gilmore, A. (Eds.) *Current Trends in British Gerontology*. Gower Press.
20. Wheatley, V. 'Relative Stress', *Community Care*, 28:8:80, 324, pp. 22-23.
21. Sanford, J.R.A. 'Tolerance of debility in elderly dependents by supporters at home: its significance for hospital practice', *British Medical Journal, 3, pp. 471-3, 1975.*
22. Challis, D. & Davies, B. 'A new approach to community care for the elderly', *British Journal of Social Work*, 10, 1, Spring 1980, pp. 1-18.
23. Gilleard, C. & Watt, G. 'The impact of day hospital care on the supporters of the elderly mentally infirm', Paper presented at the British Gerontological Society Conference, Aberdeen, 1980.
24. Fuller, J., Ward, E., Evans, A., Massam, K. & Gardner, A. 'Dementia: supportive groups for relatives' in *British Medical Journal*, 1, 1979, pp.684-5.
25. Crosbie, D. 'A role for anyone? A description of social work with the elderly in two area offices'. *British Journal of Social Work*, 13, 2 April 1983, 123-147.
26. Levin, E, Sinclair, I. and Gorbach, P. 'Supporters of Confused Elderly Persons at Home'. Extracts from main research report. Available from National Institute for Social Work, Mary Ward House, 5/7 Tavistock Place, London WC1. Price £2.

A Model of Practice in Field Care

Norma Macleod & Malcolm Smith

INTRODUCTION

This paper is an attempt to draw together ideology, practice and evaluation in care of the elderly in the Western Isles. In compiling the paper we were aware that each of the three concepts while separate in themselves are intertwined in the practice of providing the service, the planning and the subsequent modifications of it. The work referred to in the paper reflects the attempts of many to provide a service to the elderly, ranging from the policy makers i.e. the elected members, to the basic grade workers and volunteers in the community. The paper as well as illustrating successes, attempts to show failures and highlight difficulties where these have occurred, and takes the whole gamut of services from community to residential care.

The Western Isles has an elderly population of 6,500 scattered over a geographic area of 1,100 square miles; the largest island being Lewis in the North and the smallest being Vatersay in the South.

The concept of community care in the Western Isles arises from direct community demand voiced in individual contact, community surveys and need expressed through Community Associations. In 1978 a particular community survey was carried out. It was a comprehensive study of the numbers of elderly and handicapped in the community, degrees of handicap, social supports and services desired. The survey was financed by the Manpower Services Commission, and every island household was visited. One of the main findings of the survey was that 90% of elderly persons hoped that when they eventually required care, they would be helped to remain in their own community as long as possible.

The Western Isles Islands Council did not find this figure altogether surprising, because it has always considered that the provision which it makes for the elderly should be geared to community care, and not necessarily based on national guidelines and implications. The council is sympathetic to the consideration of any new proposals for care of the elderly and is constantly eager to extend its learning and experience of new approaches. Many members know from direct experience what care of the elderly is about and that family and community networks are to be supported in the giving of it. The Council therefore encourages a policy that each case is taken individually, and is moving more and more towards providing a service to the elderly to suit local needs and based on community patterns hitherto established, rather than reflecting national norms.

As with all authorities however, central government dictates still determine how finance is allocated. It is not too difficult to get capital consent to build institutions for the care of the elderly. Such capital can amount to millions of pounds, with authorities involved in heavy loan charges and running costs. No equivalent sum is available to be allocated to finance community services for the elderly, even although the community itself is quite clear as to its preference for such forms of care.

It would be fascinating to see what kind of programmes for community as opposed to institutional care of the elderly would be prepared and implemented by local authorities if finance were allocated centrally for the purpose.

WESTERN ISLES COMMUNITY SOCIAL WORK SERVICES

The ageing population in the islands is part of a strong family network. The vast majority of elderly persons as in most other local authority areas are looked after at home either by relatives who have moved in with their elderly members or who have houses close by. The current elderly population, probably more than any other, has witnessed a vast change in the community during their own lifetime, and a sense of responsibility is felt towards them by the younger generation.

Although many elderly people stay with their families, these families require environmental supports. Some families may well be able to cope but caring without respite for an elderly person over many years can tax strong as well as slender family resources.

In providing a service for the elderly person and his family social work departments require an understanding not only of the ageing process and its many concomitants but of the wider social structure of which the elderly population forms a branch.

Planning of services for the elderly must take place against the backcloth of the values of the wider community and these services developed according to community ethos. Ideally no solution to a problem, no matter how strange it may initially seem, should be discarded.

In the Western Isles we believe that families who support their elderly should themselves be supported. Such families can, through this approach, feel enabled to go on with their caring task, and the provision of a home help for an hour per day to a family to enable them to continue caring for the further twenty-three hours of the day, is a very small price to pay in comparison to admission to a residential home.

The two main factors that bring services to the elderly to a greater prominence than perhaps occur in other areas are firstly, the numbers of elderly in the community and secondly, the scattered rural nature of much of the Western Isles. These have a heightened effect on demand for services for the elderly and make difficult some solutions such as day care, but also give opportunities for a fresh look at service provision.

The percentage of the total population aged 65 and over is given in the following chart:

Area	Aged 65 - 74	Aged 75 +
Scotland	8.7%	4.3%
Western Isles	11.19%	8.08%

While comparison of the Western Isles figure for the 65 - 74 year olds shows a significant increase over the Scottish average figure, those aged 75 and over are almost twice the average rate.

The home help service

The main community service provided by the social work department to the elderly is the Home Help Service.

Frequently in the Western Isles clients are encouraged to choose their own home help from the list of those available in their community. This means that clients, if they so wish, can have as their home help somebody who is already meaningful to them both in their past history and in their current social context. Because of this, the home help and the client merely formalise what has been for many years a personal relationship. Consequently the home help takes a personal responsibility for her client, and often she is the first person on the scene at times of crisis. Clients without immediate family ties have been known to have round the clock attention from their home help, even sometimes being moved in with the home help's family during periods of illness. Husbands of home helps often play a large part in the Home Help Service in that they clean chimneys and carry out other odd jobs for their wives' clients. Elderly clients sometimes act as grandparents to their home help's children and home helps frequently bring their clients a share of any family treats.

The basing of the Home Help Service in this way on existing community informal relationships has proved to be the main resource for the elderly and their families needing support, because it oversteps the bounds of the formal contact, a concept more associated with city life.

The Scottish average provision is 9.3 home helps per 1000 total population, a figure which rises to 20.05 in the Western Isles. This is partly accounted for by the greater proportion of elderly people in the community. Another reason is that Meals on Wheels were not a viable proposition outwith Stornoway, and where elderly and isolated people might in another setting be provided with Meals on Wheels, the Home Help Service is, in the rural areas, more economic to provide and a more effective antidote to loneliness. It is for straight forward reasons such as these that the nationally issued Department of Health and Social Security Guidelines of provision for the elderly mean very little in the local context of the Western Isles.

The Department of Health and Social Security provision of 12 home helps per 1000 population over 65 compares with 21.7 per 1000 population over 65 in the Western Isles, while the Department of Health and Social Security Guidelines of 200 meals per 1000 population compares with no service of this kind in the Western Isles community.

In describing the impact of the Home Help Service on the community, it is important to note that four out of five home helps have a one-to-one relationship with their client; in other words they are not employed in more than one household. The Scottish statistics show that on average each home help has over three clients even in a comparable rural area such as parts of Highland Region.

The effect of the one-to-one relationship between home help and client is one of the most significant factors in the way the Home Help Service provides personal care and attention for many elderly people in the community. It not only provides a more comprehensive service than informal community supports but often creates a relationship that provides a client, who might not necessarily receive community support, with the kind of assistance that they desperately require.

Mrs. MacL, an elderly widow who suffers from paranoid delusions exaggerated by poor sight, lived a very isolated and lonely existence because her behaviour problems tended to make people in the community shy away from her. After a great deal of persuasion she accepted a home help and was fortunate enough to be offered the assistance of a young housewife who was able to separate those aspects of her client's behaviour attributable to illness rather than personal animosity. In this kind of case, without the formal input of a home help, it is unlikely that any person offering assistance would remain in contact with Mrs. MacL. long enough to make the distinction the home help was able to in this case.

Now we have Mrs. MacL. enjoying not only the regular support and assistance of the Home Help Service, but also the informal additions of Christmas dinner and visits to the home help's household.

Although these major benefits arise from the one-to-one relationship, this ratio is largely an accident of geography rather than a deliberate policy of encouraging more personal contact between the home help and the client. While the Home Help Organiser's task in the urban area is to assess the requirements of a client and look up the books for a suitable registered home help, in rural areas the Organiser's task also involves individual recruitment of home helps for cases, sometimes at the suggestion of the client.

In order to evaluate this major community service, there is, for the vast majority of home help clients, a twice yearly joint review of each case between the Home Help Organisers and the Community Nursing staff for each area. At these reviews the current provision for each client is assessed, and in the light of the preceding home visit by the Organiser, and the medical information provided by the nursing staff, the hours allocated to a client may be varied. Quite apart from giving more comprehensive information on which to base an accurate assessment, this system provides the nursing services with an understanding that the home help budget has limits, and that it is in the best interest of clients if the nursing staff keep us up to date with new medical information which can influence the allocation of hours according to need.

Evening care

This form of care is, at the moment, experimental.

When a local charitable trust offered a modest sum of money for the benefit of the elderly and handicapped within the town of Stornoway, with the purpose of preventing residential care, it was suggested that a visiting/auxiliary nursing service could be provided for elderly people who require personal attention in the late evening. It has long been recognised that a grey area exists between the duties of the Home Help Service and the Nursing Service, and it is hoped that, on an experimental basis, this new service will be provided to clients within the town of Stornoway. The functions of evening care assistance will range from helping clients to get ready for bed to preparing hot water bottles, to toileting, and on some occasions purely for social contact.

If for instance this kind of care were offered to Mrs. MacL. to supplement the Home Help Service, it would prove beneficial, because one of the problems the community has had to cope with is that she could hardly ever be guaranteed to prepare herself for bed and often wandered the streets in the late evening. An evening care assistant could help Mrs. MacL. prepare for bed which, is both a service to her and a very direct service to her anxious immediate community.

Domiciliary care assistant

Any style of social services which is expanding into new areas has its setbacks and the first attempt at providing domiciliary full-time care assistance to handicapped clients cannot be said to have been a success.

In this case, the clients are not elderly, but had the service proved successful it would undoubtedly have been considered for elderly couples.

A and M, a brother and sister suffer from a severe muscular complaint which has seriously limited mobility to the point where residential care appeared imperative. The problem, apart from finding suitable accommodation, was that these clients were very attached to the isolated community in which they lived and had no intention of leaving it.

As an alternative to residential care, because we appreciated the importance of their being attached to their community, a full-time Care Assistant was employed based in their house, where there was adequate sleeping-in accommodation. The formality of the arrangement seems, in some ways, to have been its downfall because it turned out in practice that the Care Assistant was on call all the time, even when in theory she was "off duty". Rules and regulations properly introduced to control the employment conditions of Care Assistants were inappropriate in an individual house and the experiment ended after three months.

It is interesting to note that in this case an informal arrangement where a retired nurse in the community now provides night care, directly employed by the clients who pay from Attendance Allowance, seems to be working very successfully.

Adaptations to houses

In order to extend the policy of encouraging elderly people to continue living at home, the Western Isles Islands Council has, under Section 12 of the Social Work (Scotland) Act, developed a scheme of assistance to elderly persons to make their houses wind and watertight, should lack of this be the main reason for their requiring care. It is appreciated that removal from what might to another person seem difficult living circumstances, can to the client be the end of the road, and consequently clients can now have repairs made to their croft houses to make them liveable, paid for through the social work department budget if this is thought to be in the best interests of the client.

The single tier structure of the authority comes into play in the implementation of this practice. The Environmental Health Department, responsible for grants under the Housing (Financial Provision) (Scotland) Act in creating housing action areas, has co-operated with the social work department in ensuring that the grants available to elderly people for modification of their houses are made use of.

In one recent case, the house of an elderly client who lived in deteriorating circumstances has been improved using in part the grants to which she is entitled under Housing Action, and in part a grant from the social work department, under Section 12, to cover the balance of the costs.

Such improvements may at first sight appear to be expensive, particularly in view of the limited budget available to the social work department for this purpose. It is undoubtedly true that public money has to be sensibly used, but when expenditure of £2,000 towards such an improvement is balanced against the current cost of £6,000 per annum for one client in a residential home, it becomes clear that a financial injection of the kind described has given the client a longer life in the community in which she wants to stay, at less cost than the option of residential care.

Relief holidays

The fact that the very expensive resource of residential care offered a facility to a relatively small proportion of the elderly population made the social work department look at the uses of such care.

It was recognised that forty beds in a residential home for the elderly can mean forty places for forty elderly in one year or alternatively, by reassigning two or three of these beds for "holiday admissions" the facility could be extended to one hundred people in one year, forty long term and sixty short term admissions.

Although it evolved from the arrangements for full residential care and applicants are screened by the same group that monitors long term admissions, the concept of relief holidays is distinct from an elderly person being received into care, and different criteria of need are applied in these cases. The holiday, of course, need not take place merely once a year and some of these beds are used by clients who come in on a number of occasions. The hope, now borne out to some extent in practice, is that by offering a regular relief holiday to an elderly person, the family will find its caring role made easier by regularly being relieved of that responsibility.

This can be illustrated in the case of Miss MacD. who had been accommodated by relatives after a period of illness. In rather overcrowded conditions she felt a burden to her relatives but physically was unable to live on her own. A number of short admissions to one of the Homes made life tolerable for Miss MacD. and her relatives and recently she was allocated the joint tenancy of a sheltered house, where she retains independence and has the assistance she requires.

In the light of the relatively recent experience of short term use of residential beds, the social work department has begun to look seriously at the extension of this policy and the senior staff in the Homes involved wish to see short term admission expanding. Their feeling is that by this expansion they could provide an effective service to a far greater number in the community and have increased job satisfaction in creating positive rehabilitation programmes as well as the more traditional types of care.

Day care

Department of Health and Social Security Guidelines on provision of social work services become rather meaningless when the concept of day care is considered within the Western Isles, because day care is a possibility only for those who live within a certain catchment area of our five residential homes. For an elderly person living in Uig to travel forty miles to Stornoway daily for day care would almost certainly counteract any beneficial effects.

Sheltered housing

The islands saw an extensive programme of sheltered housing developed during the 1970s. In 1975, at the inception of the Western Isles Islands Council, no modern schemes were in existence although a number were about to be built. There are now fourteen sheltered housing schemes in operation with warden and alarm facilities, and assessment of need for further schemes is frequently taking place. The schemes are all very small, the largest being in a rural area and comprising twelve houses. Normally schemes range from 6 - 12 houses and in some areas are as small as four houses.

In the rural communities sheltered housing has quickly assumed popularity among the elderly population and despite being a new concept to the elderly, who are traditionally slow to accept change, the sheltered housing programme is seen to be a considerable success.

As the warden service is provided by the social work department and the houses managed by the housing department, there has to exist a co-operation between the two departments. Allocation of the houses, while having to operate within the normal rules of housing management, is almost totally at the discretion of the social work department.

In one of the schemes, rather different from the others in that it is a physical part of one of the Homes for the elderly, the "very sheltered" nature of the housing has led to it being used and allocated on a different basis to other sheltered housing and it has virtually become a direct social work resource. From this housing arises real prospects of rehabilitation of long term residents to a sort of independence, where a move to the "outside world" would be too much to contemplate. Old friendships from the Home can be retained, and daily use of common rooms between areas need not make the move too dramatic. The availability of housing of this kind to promote rehabilitation work must presuppose a close and purposeful relationship between social work and housing departments.

The introduction of new concepts, however well researched, is always a bit of a hit and miss affair, and the appending of a Tigh Ceilidh (communal meeting room) to sheltered housing schemes is an example of this. The Tigh Ceilidh was conceived as an opportunity for the mainly elderly residents to get together in a warm comfortable place to counteract the possible loneliness of independent living. However, residents have largely avoided using this facility. Some see it as being quite unnatural to meet their friends anywhere but by their own or by their friends' firesides, which is the private and traditional place where people visit or "ceilidh" with one another. In retrospect the addition of the Tigh Ceilidh for the use of the elderly was perhaps rather an artificial and clinical recreation of the past, but these are gradually now becoming community facilities geared to the needs of other groups who are more attuned to meeting socially in such places. It is likely because of this that future generations of elderly people may be more active in their use of the Tigh Ceilidh.

Care units

An interesting innovation in rural care of the elderly has been the establishing of Care Units as part of Sheltered Housing Schemes in the more remote rural areas. This development is based on the fact that the Council acknowledged that all its residential facilities were based in the centres of population, thus requiring admissions to be made from areas of up to 40 miles distance. Such a process means that relatives of elderly persons find it difficult to travel regularly to such centres to keep in touch with their elderly relatives, and that the influence of the elderly is being lost to particular communities.

Care Units were developed from the basic plans for sheltered housing, being constructed as two sheltered houses linked together with a common living room. The Units are linked to the normal alarm system of the sheltered housing but night care within the Unit can be made available if required. Four persons can be accommodated in the Unit. The sheltered housing warden has overall responsibility for the Unit's functioning, embracing care and administration, with input from other part time staff as required.

The Council policy for Care Units is that within them care should be provided for various categories of persons and not merely be regarded as a small version of an Old Persons Home.

Even in such small establishments, in a relatively short time, institutional modes of coping begin to manifest themselves, both among residents and staff and unless a clear policy of admission, discharge, and staff supplementation is in evidence, the wider community tends to see the Unit either as an Old Persons Home or Geriatric Hospital.

Attendant on the development of Care Units in rural areas should be the development of day care, hitherto unavailable except in areas close to residential homes.

Residential homes

As in all authorities a tiny percentage of Western Isles elderly live in residential homes. Some of these Homes can, like many such places, be institutional in nature, and in support to staff, programmes have to be initiated to give the resident a sense of community.

To this end one of our Homes was recently upgraded to create small kitchen/sitting areas similar to the typical island kitchen, to encourage residents to prepare breakfasts, to clean up, and have visitors on their own terms.

The rehabilitation process here is long and hard and we need to have much more understanding of environmental effects upon people.

The whole policy on residential care provided by the social work department has strong links with Health Board facilities, at Stornoway, Daliburgh and Barra.

The screening group which monitors admission to the Lewis Homes has in its membership the consultant geriatrician and, in turn, the admission meeting to the geriatric hospital in Stornoway, held each week has social work representation. In this way ''clients'' referred for residential and hospital care can be looked upon as a group and more appropriate assistance offered than where nominal or no cross information or referral exists. The other effect of this co-operation is that a trust develops between the various professional workers and a greater understanding exists of the boundaries of each discipline and what it can appropriately offer.

The most recently built residential establishment is a fifteen-bedded Home in North Uist, different in design from our more traditional buildings. The establishment comprises three separate buildings, and a Tigh Ceilidh which incorporates minimum residential facilities for night care staff. The three buildings are similar in type to Care Units, and are geared towards small scale community living. There are no long corridors and the buildings have deliberately not been linked together, in order to encourage residents to go outside should they wish to visit a resident in another part of the building. This enables residents to continue what is normal visiting practice from their own home, and to continue facing reasonable outdoor risks.

The operational philosophy underlying the proposals, as in the establishing of Care Units, is the goal of helping to minimise residents' dependence on staff, an extremely hard task which is only partly related to building design.

It is difficult to know how institutional modes of coping set in, and they are of course linked to a number of factors such as the elderly person's view of authority which will be traditional, (i.e. not realising that the new environment is theirs to manipulate) and a wish to be a 'good' resident. It may also be to do with the fact that although we are designing buildings geared to support residents' efforts to care for themselves and counter the institutional effects of traditionally designed Homes, we have not yet been able to take the step in helping staff who are largely untrained to carry out the caring task to fit in with the philosophy.

CONCLUSION

While it is possible to show the thread of a developing policy that runs through these services, namely to shape provision to the community it serves, it would not be correct to present an account of provision in a way that suggested a unitary approach, either in philosophy or real service.

The reality is that services are based on legislation spanning the twentieth century, buildings which fall out of step with developments in and approaches to care of the elderly, and staff whose training and attitudes may match the span of legislation.

Developments in joint planning with the Western Isles Health Board over the years have enabled the Council to go ahead with the projects mentioned and a number of them have enjoyed and are still enjoying the benefits of support and financing.

When such joint work proves to be effective between two statutory bodies it is to be regretted that the possibility exists of support financing being available in the future on a population basis only rather than on giving due weight to rural deprivation, demographic and distance factors which have considerable effect on the range of services required in an area such as the Western Isles. Distribution on a population basis only is more than likely to mean that the Council would not be able to finance further innovations in the community.

Other Information

New literature on old age is compiled by the Centre for Policy on Ageing, for the busy professional who needs to keep up-to-date with the subject. This bulletin, published every two months, is a guide to current books, government reports and circulars, pamphlets and periodical articles on ageing and related issues. It covers both British and relevant overseas publications. Also included is a section devoted to forthcoming courses, conferences and meetings of interest to the readership. The 1985 subscription (6 issues) is £12.00.

Old age: a register of social research provides a detailed description of current or recently completed research projects on ageing and old age. Like *New literature on old age*, it covers such issues as health and health services, psychology, the sociology of ageing and every aspect of social policy for older age groups. The register is published by the Centre for Policy on Ageing for all who need to be up-to-date with research, or to identify 'who's who' in British age research. The 1980/81 edition (published March 1982) costs £12.00 plus postage.

Further details for both publications from:
Centre for Policy on Ageing
Nuffield Lodge Studio
Regent's Park
London NW1 4RS
Telephone 01 586 9844

Order from Bailey Brothers and Swinfen Ltd., Warner House, Folkestone, Kent CT19 6PH.

Centre for Policy on Ageing also maintains Britain's only reference major *library* on ageing and old age, which is open to the public. For details, please contact CPA at Nuffield Lodge Studio, Regent's Park, London NW1 4RS. Telephone 01 586 9844.

British Society of Gerontology was established in 1973 to provide a multidisciplinary forum for researchers in the field of ageing. Its aim is to encourage research and study of human ageing and later life and application of this knowledge to the improvement of the quality of life. Members of the Society are drawn principally from the social and behavioural sciences and the humanities; and include researchers and members of the caring professions. The Society's interests span theoretical studies, empirical investigations, methodological issues and policy analyses relevant not only to older people but to ageing throughout the whole life span.

The Society's main activities are the provision of media for the exchange of information and ideas which take the form of conferences, seminars and publications. The annual conference held in a different location each September is the main event. It includes plenary sessions and workshops run simultaneously on a number of different themes so as to provide for the wide range of interests represented in the Society. BSG publishes a regular bulletin for members *Ageing Times* and occasional reports, primarily conference proceedings. The Society's journal *Ageing and Society* is published four times a year by Cambridge University Press.

Details of membership may be obtained from the Secretary of the Society, Dr. A.M. Warnes, Department of Geography, King's College, University of London, The Strand, London WC2.

The Age Concern Research Unit was established in 1975 and is based at Age Concern England's headquarters. It has conducted a major national survey of people aged 75 and over and has produced a series of reviews of existing research information in the form of *Profiles on the Elderly:* who the elderly are, their standards of living and life satisfaction, their health, their welfare and use of the personal social services, accidents and their mobility. Age Concern England has published several of the reports produced by the Unit and has made use of research material in a variety of ways.

The Research Unit is currently engaged on a study of the values of older people and another on the needs and circumstances of elders in ethnic minorities as well as on a longitudinal study following up people who were aged 65 to 69 when first interviewed. It has initiated a programme of action research and monitoring and evaluation of certain services, especially of new initiatives in the care of elderly people or the support of their relatives. It is also seeking funds to enable it to conduct research on processes of becoming ''housebound'', sources and value of friendship in later life, children's images of old people and hospital and community psychogeriatric services in two health districts. It is expected that all these studies will have important implications for education and for the design and delivery of services.

Further details of the work of the Unit can be obtained from:
Jonathan Baker
Age Concern Research Unit
60 Pitcairn Road
Mircham
Surrey CR4 3LL
Telephone 01 640 5431